KING of POISONS

Related Titles from Potomac Books

*Man and Wound in the Ancient World: A History of Military Medicine
from Sumer to the Fall of Constantinople*
—Richard A. Gabriel

*Between Flesh and Steel: A History of Military Medicine
from the Middle Ages to the War in Afghanistan*
—Richard A. Gabriel

KING of POISONS

A HISTORY OF ARSENIC

JOHN PARASCANDOLA

Potomac Books
An imprint of the University of Nebraska Press

Library of Congress Cataloging-in-Publication Data
Parascandola, John, 1941–
    King of poisons : a history of arsenic / John Parascandola. — 1st ed.
        p. ; cm.
    Includes bibliographical references and index.
    ISBN 978-1-59797-703-6 (cloth : alk. paper)
    ISBN 978-1-59797-809-5 (e-book)
    I. Title.
    [DNLM: 1. Arsenic Poisoning—history. 2. Arsenic—therapeutic use. 3. History of Medicine. QV 294]
        615.9'25715—dc23

                                                                    2012028480

Printed on acid-free paper that meets the American National Standards Institute Z39-48 Standard.

First Edition

To my parents-in-law,
Roslyn and Daniel Weisberg

Contents

Acknowledgments   ix

Introduction   I

1   King of Poisons: *Arsenic and Murder*   5

2   Poison in the Plot: *Arsenic in Fiction*   53

3   Hazards on the Job: *Arsenic in the Workplace*   83

4   The Ubiquitous Element: *Arsenic in the Environment*   109

5   What Kills Can Cure: *Arsenic in Medicine*   145

Suggested Further Readings   173

Notes   175

Index   193

About the Author   199

Acknowledgments

Years ago, while conducting research in the history of pharmacology and toxicology, I became fascinated with the history of arsenic. I have long wanted to write a book on the subject for a broad audience. This book is aimed more toward the general reader than to the specialist in the history of medicine and science, although scholars in these and related fields looking for an overview of the subject should find it useful as well.

The book is based on an extensive number and wide variety of secondary and primary sources. I am indebted to many previous authors on the subject. The works cited in the list of suggested further readings were especially useful. The sources for the images in the book are gratefully acknowledged in the captions.

Many people contributed suggestions or comments in connection with my research and writing, and I cannot list them all. However, I would like to acknowledge and thank several individuals who were especially helpful. My brother, Louis Parascandola, brought to my attention a number of literary works that featured arsenic as part of the story. My editor at Potomac Books, Elizabeth Demers, read the manuscript and made many useful suggestions for changes. I also wish to thank two other members of the Potomac Books staff, Amanda Irle, who guided me through the copyediting process, and Liz Norris, whose copyediting significantly improved the manuscript. Last, but certainly not least, I wish to express my appreciation to my wife, Randee, for her support and encouragement throughout this project.

Introduction

The very name of arsenic conjures up images of murder and intrigue. It is in many ways the quintessential poison and was for centuries undoubtedly the most frequently used substance for the purpose of homicide. In the words of John Emsley, "Arsenic has a long and disreputable pedigree: its very name seems to condemn it as something unspeakable."[1] The word itself has a complicated history but ultimately seems to go back to the Greek word *arsenikon*, meaning "bold" or "potent."

Arsenic trioxide, also called arsenic oxide, is the form in which the element was most commonly administered in cases of murder, and frequently it is this compound that people were actually describing when they referred to arsenic. The oxide is colorless, odorless, and tasteless, and dissolves readily in water and other liquids. It is thus not easy for the victim to detect that he or she is being poisoned. As it is a cumulative poison, small doses can be given over a long period of time, eventually killing someone without necessarily arousing suspicion. The prominent gastrointestinal effects of arsenic were easily mistaken for diseases that were common throughout much of history, such as cholera. Also, there weren't any good tests for detecting arsenic in body tissues until well into the nineteenth century.

Clearly, it is arsenic's poisonous properties that have most fascinated the public over time. However, even this part of the story goes well beyond arsenic's criminal uses. Countless individuals over the centuries have been the victims of unintentional poisoning with arsenic, especially in more modern times. Arsenic is much more than a poison used to dispatch one's enemies or those who get in one's way. Arsenic has had many commercial uses that made it a common substance in the workplace and the environment, especially

I

beginning in the nineteenth century. Arsenic's value as a green pigment, for example, led to its inclusion in wallpaper, paint, fabrics, and other common domestic items, exposing both the workers who produced these products and the consumers who purchased them to possible poisoning. Arsenic also had numerous other industrial uses, including as a pesticide and as a preservative. In addition, although it may seem odd given its poisonous reputation, arsenic has been used as a medicine since ancient times.

This book tells the fascinating story of arsenic in its many aspects. It begins by looking at arsenic's history as an intentional poison. Given its common use for this purpose throughout much of recorded history, arsenic has often been labeled the King of Poisons. The first chapter examines this murderous history. Not surprisingly, arsenic has been frequently used for homicidal purposes in fiction as well as in real life, and the second chapter will cover the history of arsenic in literature. The focus next turns to unintentional poisoning, looking first at arsenic poisoning in the workplace and then in the broader environment. The final chapter deals with the use of arsenic in medicine.

To begin with, however, some general information about arsenic is in order. Arsenic is an element with the symbol As, an atomic number of 33, and an atomic mass of 74.9. It is classified in Group 15 of the periodic table, along with nitrogen, phosphorous, antimony, and bismuth. The first two of these elements are nonmetals, and the last two are metals. Arsenic falls in the middle of this group and is considered a metalloid (i.e., it has properties of both metals and nonmetals, although it is frequently called a metal).

Estimates of arsenic's concentration in the Earth's crust range from about 1 to 5 parts per million, meaning that it is not one of the more abundant terrestrial elements. But it is concentrated in some parts of the Earth due to its close association with certain other metals and due to human activities such as mining and pesticide manufacture. It also occurs in air and water, generally in small amounts, but again can be concentrated in certain areas, creating toxicity problems. For example, the high arsenic content of drinking water in Bangladesh and West Bengal, India, is poisoning millions of people today. William Cullen has noted that "the U.S. Agency for Toxic Substances and Disease Registry (ATSDR) ranks arsenic as No. 1 on its list of priority hazardous substances because of both its prevalence in contaminated environments and its toxicity. This ranking has not changed for many years."[2]

Arsenic is rarely found as an element in nature but usually occurs in the forms of the sulfide compounds orpiment (As_2S_3) and realgar (As_4S_4), or as the iron-sulfur compound arsenopyrite (FeAsS). When heated in air, it combines with oxygen to form arsenic trioxide (As_2O_3), which is the most toxic form of arsenic. Although arsenic exists in nature largely in the form of such inorganic compounds, the element can also bind to organic (i.e., carbon-containing) compounds. Many organic arsenic compounds have been synthesized and used as medicines and for other purposes. Organic arsenic compounds are generally less toxic than inorganic compounds of the element.

Some studies suggest that arsenic may be essential to animals and even humans, although the evidence is not definitive enough yet to establish this with certainty. Recently, controversy has also developed over a claim by a team of researchers led by Felisa Wolfe-Simon of the NASA Astrobiology Institute (NAI) that they had discovered a species of bacteria that substituted arsenic for the phosphorous usually used to build DNA, the basic genetic material of living organisms. The idea of arsenic-based life challenges the understanding of the basic requirements of life held by scientists in general, and the study has been criticized by some as being deficient and drawing unjustified conclusions. As this book was going to press, the journal *Science*, based on two new studies, stated that the original Wolfe-Simon paper that it had published was incorrect in some of its major findings and that arsenic did not substitute for phosphorous in the bacterium. Wolfe-Simon and her coworkers, however, defended their original conclusions.[3]

Arsenic thus remains a subject of controversy today, as it has throughout its history. Whether as a poison or a medicine, a pesticide or a preservative, or for whatever purpose it was used, arsenic has been viewed as a blessing and a curse. Of course, it is neither, merely a chemical element. How we use it determines whether it helps or harms. A doctor can use arsenic trioxide to cure someone suffering from acute promyelocytic leukemia (APL), or a murderer can slip it into someone's coffee. In this book, we shall examine essentially all aspects of the riveting history of this most famous of poisons. We shall explore the many purposes to which arsenic has been put over the ages and better understand why it is the King of Poisons.

CHAPTER ONE

King of Poisons
Arsenic and Murder

Who discovered the poisonous properties of arsenic, and who first used it to murder a fellow human? The answers to these questions are lost to history. The naturally occurring arsenic sulfides realgar and orpiment were known in ancient times and were even used to some extent in medicine. The fact that they were toxic was certainly recognized, but they would not have been useful for homicidal purposes. These compounds are insoluble and colored, and so would have been difficult to administer to someone undetected. The form in which arsenic is generally used as a poison is arsenic trioxide, a white powder that has sometimes been called white arsenic. The trioxide dissolves readily in water and is colorless and tasteless, thus making it an ideal poison. The poisonous nature of arsenic trioxide and methods for making the compound, which does not occur in nature, were certainly known by the ancient Greeks and Romans. It is easily produced, for example, by the smelting of copper ores that contain arsenic as an impurity. Roasting orpiment would also produce a white compound that would have been largely arsenic trioxide. The sodium salt of the trioxide, which had similar properties to the trioxide, could be prepared readily by heating orpiment with natural sodium carbonate.

Some accounts argue that arsenic trioxide was the poison used by Agrippina the Younger and her son, Nero, to eliminate his rivals for emperor of Rome. The evidence for such a claim, however, is not definitive, and other substances, such as cyanide, are also possible candidates. Plants, such as hemlock and wolfsbane, were apparently the most widely used poisons in ancient Greece and Rome. Hemlock, of course, was the poison administered by the city-state of Athens to execute Socrates, and wolfsbane was actually so frequently used as a poison that the emperor Trajan banned the growing of the plant in Roman domestic gardens.[1]

It was not until the beginning of the fifteenth century that arsenic became popular as a poison. The most notorious name associated with poisoning in the Italian Renaissance period is the Borgia family, especially Rodrigo Borgia (who became Pope Alexander VI in 1492) and two of his children, Cesare and Lucrezia. It appears that Lucrezia has become unfairly associated with murder, however, as exemplified by the scene in Donizetti's opera *Lucrezia Borgia* where she poisons five people. In reality, Lucrezia was a pious woman who died at the age of 39, probably without poisoning anyone. There seems to be little doubt of the guilt of her father and brother, however. Cesare, in particular, probably poisoned dozens of people in the furtherance of political ends. Arsenic (probably the trioxide) was almost certainly the key ingredient in the Borgias' favorite poison, called La Cantarella.

Poisoning became a formal method of assassination in Italy. By the six-teenth century, there was a branch of the government of Venice that arranged for the elimination of enemies of the state. Professional poisoners worked for hire and charged fees. In Naples, beginning in the second half of the sev-enteenth century, a woman named Giulia Toffana (La Toffana) gained noto-riety as a poisoner. Arsenic appears to have been the crucial ingredient in the poison she sold, which was frequently referred to as Aqua Toffana. When La Toffana was finally arrested and executed in 1709, she confessed (probably under torture, so the reliability of her information is questionable) to being responsible for the poisoning of some six hundred people. In the mid-sixteenth century, another woman named Hieronyma Spara (La Spara) sold an arsenic-based poison in Rome. La Spara even formed a society where she taught women how to get rid of their husbands with the use of poison.[2]

Catherine de Medici (who married Henry II, the future king of France, in 1533) often gets the credit for bringing the Italian art of poisoning to France and using it for political gain, although this view has not gone unchallenged.[3] There was a widespread belief in France that Italians were a devious people who got rid of their enemies by covert means. Italians were deemed experts on poisons, possessing secret knowledge of powerful toxins.

The French were themselves making significant use of arsenic and other poisons for political or personal gain by the seventeenth century. Marie-

Madeleine-Marguérite d'Aubray, marquise de Brinvilliers, was notorious for murdering members of her family to gain wealth and property in the second half of the century. She reputedly tested out her poisonous concoctions (which included arsenic) on hapless patients in a hospital in Paris, mixing the poison in the gifts of food and drink that she brought for the sick, although most likely this story is a myth. Her crimes were eventually discovered, and she was beheaded in 1676.

Another famous French poisoner of that period was Catherine Deshayes Monvoisin (La Voisin). When her husband went bankrupt, La Voisin supported her family by carrying out abortions, performing witchcraft, and selling love potions and poisons. Arsenic appears to have been a main ingredient in one of her poisons. Convicted of involvement in poisoning and abortion, she was tortured and burned at the stake. Poisoning had become so common in the court of Louis XIV that the king, convinced he himself was in danger, established a special commission to investigate the matter. By the time the commission finished its work in 1682, its investigation had led to the trial of 104 persons, 34 of whom were executed, with others receiving sentences of banishment or imprisonment. A royal edict issued in that year decreed that anyone convicted of supplying poison for the purpose of murder, whether or not the act resulted in fatalities, would be subject to the death penalty.[4]

The British also tended to view poisoning as particularly associated with Italy. They even referred to the act of poisoning as "Italianation," but such crimes occurred in Britain as well. By the sixteenth century, court records reveal that trials involving poisoning were occurring regularly, if not frequently. One source recorded a dozen criminal poisonings between 1571 and 1598. Not surprisingly, arsenic was one of the weapons of choice for British poisoners. In 1712 servant Elizabeth Mason used arsenic in an attempt to murder the two women who employed her. One woman died, but the other survived, and the servant was hanged.[5]

The evidence suggests that poisoning probably reached a peak in England in the mid-nineteenth century (although poisoning was still much less frequent than other means of homicidal violence). By far the most common poison for homicide was arsenic. In a study of 540 English criminal poisoning cases between 1750 and 1914, Katherine Watson found that arsenic (in the form of the oxide or the sulfides) was involved in 237 cases. The next most common poison, opium, was a distant second, involved in 52 cases. Watson commented, "The story of poisoning in England and Wales is in many ways a chronicle of the rise and fall of arsenic."[6]

Before 1851 there were no legal restrictions on the sale of poisons in England, so they were not difficult to obtain. It was especially easy to purchase arsenic. White arsenic was relatively cheap and was widely available, as it was commonly used to kill rats and other vermin. Arsenic was also used in medicine, such as in the popular medication known as Fowler's solution.[7]

Although the press tended to focus attention on high-profile poisoning cases involving people of higher social status, such as physicians and middle-class women, Watson has shown that, at least in England, poisoning was primarily a crime of the poor and underprivileged. People in unhappy or abusive marriages sometimes murdered their spouses because they were unable to get divorced if they were not wealthy. Parents might murder children because they could not afford to feed and care for them, and desperate or greedy individuals might poison a relative to reap the rewards of an insurance policy. The motives for murder were many and varied.[8]

Poison was typically viewed in the Victorian era as a woman's weapon. The poisoner was linked with characteristics stereotypically associated with women, such as secrecy and cunning. In the 540 poisoning cases studied by Watson, however, men and women were about equally represented (49 percent to 51 percent respectively) among the accused poisoners. Watson does go on to point out that these figures must be considered in light of the more general statistics concerning violent crime. Men comprised a substantial majority of those tried for murder in this period. Watson concludes, "Roughly speaking, then, men were three times more likely than women to commit murder, but women who did so were far more likely than men to choose poison as their weapon." Reviewing cases from England in the 1840s, Ian Burney found that in 60 percent of the cases, the accused party was a woman, 37 percent of whom were charged with poisoning their spouses. He also noted that in nearly 70 percent of these cases, the poison used was arsenic.[9]

Detection of Arsenic

The number of poisoning cases reported was no doubt significantly lower than the actual number of cases, at least up into the nineteenth century. There weren't any good chemical tests for most poisons, and the symptoms of poisoning were often confused with those of disease. Arsenic poisoning was particularly difficult to detect. Its symptoms were similar to those of cholera and dysentery, and there was no reliable chemical test for arsenic until the nineteenth century. Convictions of arsenic poisoning were generally based on confessions or circumstantial evidence (e.g., the accused was known to have purchased the poison and had the opportunity and motive to commit the crime).[10]

The first known case in which convincing scientific proof of poisoning was given in court took place in Oxford, England, in 1752. The accused was Mary Blandy, a thirty-one-year-old woman who was charged with poisoning her father with arsenic. Blandy had had an affair with a Scottish army officer named William Cranstoun. Mary's father learned that Cranstoun was married, although the latter denied it, and forbade her from seeing him. Cranstoun apparently believed that Mary was to inherit a large sum of money and was determined not to give her up. After returning to Scotland, he sent Mary a white powder to give to her father, telling her that it would make him more favorably disposed to their marriage. Mary administered the powder to her father in food and drink and he became seriously ill. Two maids who had eaten some of the same food also suffered some ill effects. When they noticed powder at the bottom of a pot of gruel, they turned the pot over to a local apothecary.

The physician called in to treat Blandy, Anthony Addington, suspected poisoning. Blandy informed the doctor that he became sick after eating the gruel. His symptoms included a painful burning in his mouth and intestinal tract, vomiting, and diarrhea, all consistent with arsenic poisoning. Addington and a chemist examined the powder from the pot that the maids had given to the apothecary. Addington testified at Mary's trial that he concluded that the white powder was arsenic on the basis of some chemical tests, which in reality were rather nonspecific. The powder had the following similar characteristics with white arsenic: it was milky white, it was gritty, the greater part of it sank to the bottom and remained undissolved in cold water, and it produced thick white fumes with a garlic smell when thrown onto a hot iron.

He added that it behaved the same way as arsenic did in a number of chemical tests involving the formation of precipitates.

Since Mary had confessed to putting the powder in her father's food, the main question for the jury was whether or not they believed her claim that she did not know it was poison. She indicated that she had accepted Cranstoun's explanation that the powder would simply make her father fonder of her lover. The jury obviously did not believe that she was telling the truth, since they quickly returned a verdict of guilty. Mary was hanged, but Cranstoun fled to France, where he died shortly thereafter.[11]

The tests available to Addington were suggestive but did not provide conclusive evidence of the presence of arsenic in cases of suspected poisoning. A more positive identification required a better chemical test. This became clear to James Marsh, a chemist at the Royal Arsenal in Woolwich, England, when he was called upon in 1832 to test for arsenic in a case of suspected murder in Plumstead. The accused was charged with murdering his grandfather. Since the grandson was known to have purchased arsenic, supposedly as a rat poison, Marsh was asked to test some coffee (which had made several people in the household, including the deceased, sick) and the stomach contents of the dead man. Marsh was able to produce a yellow precipitate, characteristic of the presence of arsenic, in the coffee, but the jury was not sufficiently impressed by this demonstration. Furthermore, he was unable to demonstrate the presence of arsenic in the stomach contents. The jury acquitted the defendant, who later admitted his guilt.

Frustrated by the acquittal, Marsh was determined to invent a more definitive test for arsenic. The procedure he developed was based on the discovery by pharmacist-chemist Carl Scheele in 1775 that when arsenic acid reacts with zinc, it produces a gaseous compound of arsenic and hydrogen known as arsine. The gas is highly toxic and smells somewhat like garlic. Marsh found that the gas leaves a film of metallic arsenic when burned or sufficiently heated. The amount of arsenic could be roughly estimated from the size of the film. Marsh's test allowed him to separate small quantities of arsenic from organic matter and to clearly show the presence of the arsenic through the film deposited. Tests involving the formation of precipitates could confirm that the film was arsenic. The Marsh test was adopted quickly in both the laboratory and the courtroom. The sensitivity of the test was

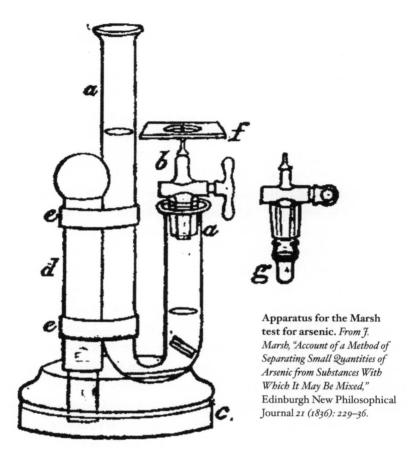

Apparatus for the Marsh test for arsenic. *From J. Marsh, "Account of a Method of Separating Small Quantities of Arsenic from Substances With Which It May Be Mixed,"* Edinburgh New Philosophical Journal *21 (1836): 229–36.*

later improved so that it could detect even smaller amounts of arsenic. The Swedish chemist Jöns Jacob Berzelius developed a quantitative version of the test in 1837. [12]

The Marsh test, however, required significant skill to perform, or the results could be erroneous or misleading. The test also took hours to complete, and it was possible to contaminate the results through the introduction of arsenic from extraneous sources. The problems involved in using the test are illustrated in the notorious trial of Marie Lafarge in France in 1840. Her husband, Charles Lafarge, died under suspicious circumstances in January 1840, and Marie was arrested and charged with poisoning him when the autopsy results suggested there was arsenic in his stomach (although the results were questionable because the test tube had exploded during the test). The world-renowned toxicologist Mathieu Orfila pointed out that there were problems with the test procedure. The court asked three chemists to repeat the test on the stomach contents and on Charles's vomit. They used the Marsh test and reported that they found no evidence of arsenic. Charles's body was exhumed and tested again, but still no arsenic was found.

The trial judge was still not satisfied, and he sent for Orfila from Paris. Convinced that Orfila's results would confirm the absence of arsenic, the defense had agreed to the reanalysis. Orfila and two of his colleagues performed the analysis and found about half a milligram of arsenic in the body and the stomach contents. In spite of the earlier results, and the relatively small amount of arsenic detected by Orfila, the jury found Marie guilty, and she was sentenced to hard labor for life (which was later commuted to just life imprisonment). She was released in 1852 after she became ill in prison.[13]

German chemist Hugo Reinsch developed a quicker and simpler test for arsenic in 1841. This test involved dipping copper foil in a boiling solution of the sample. If the sample contained arsenic, a grey material consisting of copper arsenide was deposited on the foil. When the copper arsenide was heated, it produced white crystals of arsenic trioxide that could be readily identified with the aid of a magnifying glass. Both the Marsh and the Reinsch tests became commonly used in inquests and trials involving suspected arsenic poisoning, making it harder for murderers to get away with their crimes.[14]

Efforts to Control the Availability of Arsenic

Although it became easier to detect the presence of arsenic in bodies and in the vehicles used to administer it by the middle of the nineteenth century, it still remained a popular choice for poisoners. For one thing, arsenic was readily available and inexpensive. The poisoner no doubt hoped that the crime would go undetected, with the symptoms being mistaken for those of an illness and no autopsy called for.

As early as 1819 in England, there was an effort to pass legislation establishing regulations for the sale of certain poisons and drugs, the focus being

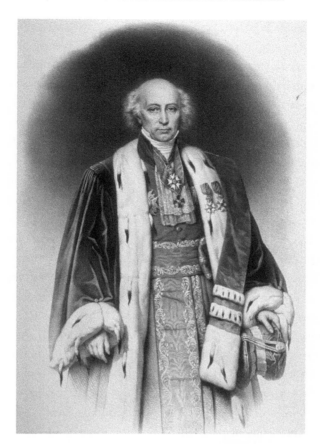

Mathieu Orfila, pioneer toxicologist, about 1815.
Courtesy of the National Library of Medicine.

on arsenic, oxalic acid, and corrosive sublimate (mercuric chloride). Druggists were concerned that the bill would interfere with the dispensing of medicines, and so they opposed it, leading to its withdrawal. The perceived increase in reported cases of poisoning in the 1840s, especially involving arsenic, prompted Parliament to revisit the issue of controlling the sale of poisons. The bill introduced was limited only to arsenic because, as stated in the preamble, "the unrestricted sale of arsenic facilitates the commission of crime." The poison was available not only in drugstores but also from grocers and other merchants.

The bill passed and became the Sale of Arsenic Regulation Act of 1851. It restricted the sale of arsenic to those over the age of twenty-one, and then only when the buyer was known to or introduced by someone known to the seller. An entry for the sale had to be made in a poison book or register and had to include the purchaser's signature. The arsenic also had to be colored with soot or indigo to make it easier to detect (although this rule did not apply to bulk sales of ten pounds or more, which were generally made to farmers, manufacturers, and wholesalers). It had originally been proposed that only males could purchase arsenic (reflecting a particular concern about female poisoners), but this provision was not included in the final bill.

Prosecutions under the act began almost immediately. In September 1851 a grocer was charged with a sale violating the act in a murder case involving arsenic. The effect of the act on poisonings in Britain, however, is debatable. Poisoners could turn to other substances for their crimes, and criminal poisoning by arsenic by no means disappeared in the years following 1851. Noted toxicologist Alfred Swaine Taylor complained in 1857 that arsenic was still cheap enough to be within the reach of even the poor and that many grocers and other shopkeepers sold the drug in an uncolored state on the most frivolous pretenses. Historian Peter Bartrip has concluded, "Given the limited terms of the Arsenic Act and the absence of effective enforcement provisions there is little reason to suppose that it exerted a significant influence upon the overall incidence of poisoning." On the other hand, fellow historian Katherine Watson believes that in spite of the piecemeal implementation of the act, it was gradually effective in reducing crimes of poisoning, especially those involving arsenic.[15]

Poisoning did become somewhat more difficult after the passage of the Pharmacy Act of 1868 (subtitled "An Act to Regulate the Sale of Poisons"). Under this law, all persons who desired to set up businesses as pharmacists or to sell "scheduled" poisons had to pass a qualifying examination administered by the Royal Pharmaceutical Society (RPS) (although those already in such a business were allowed to continue subject to certification to that effect and provided they were deemed suitable for registration). A schedule of poisons to be included under the act was also established, with the RPS having the authority to amend it. A further step was taken in the 1880s, when more zealous prosecution of illegal sales involving uncolored arsenic was initiated. However, the uncolored substance was legally present in large quantities at dye-makers, glass factories, wholesalers, and farms. In spite of these efforts, arsenic murders were not completely eliminated.[16]

In the American colonies, the only mention of poisons in legislation was in connection with using these substances for criminal purposes. A Massachusetts law of 1641, for example, stipulated that killing an individual by poisoning was punishable by death. It was not until the nineteenth century that efforts were made to exert some kind of control over the sale of poisons in the United States. Beginning with a New York law in 1829, a number of states required poisons to be conspicuously labeled as such. The first state to require that a record be kept of poison sales was New Hampshire in 1848. The American Pharmaceutical Association (APhA), which was established in 1852 and is now known as the American Pharmacists Association, recognized that the unrestricted sale of poisons in pharmacies was a "serious evil" and worked to try to safeguard the use of poisons from its founding. Most states passed pharmacy practice acts requiring the licensing of pharmacists in the last quarter of the nineteenth century, and these laws generally included restrictions on the sale of poisons. Some individuals, such as pharmacist Martin Wilbert, argued for the passage of a uniform national poison law to deal with the problem of the different nature and scope of the laws of various states, but no federal legislation was enacted, although federal laws were passed in the twentieth century restricting the sale of specific chemicals that could have poisonous effects (e.g., controlled substances such as narcotics.)[17]

Wilbert pointed out the importance and the difficulty of controlling the sale of poisons, which he believed in 1914 were being increasingly used for homicidal and suicidal purposes:

> It is generally recognized that the underlying object of legislation to control the sale and use of poisons is the protection of the public. It is practically impossible to make poison regulations foolproof, and it is also admittedly impracticable to dissuade the person bent on self-destruction from accomplishing his end. Easy access to poisons greatly increases their abuse, and it is difficult indeed to conceive of ways that will tend to prevent or even discourage the constantly growing abuse of poisonous substances.[18]

Famous Arsenic Murder Cases

Arsenic has probably been the most frequently used poison for homicidal purposes, and it is not possible to provide a comprehensive history of the subject. I have, however, selected a number of famous arsenic murder cases for discussion, some of which involve the murder of one individual and some of which involve multiple murders.

Individual Murder

GEORGE WYTHE SWEENEY[19]

In their new nation's formative years, Americans were shocked by the apparent murder of one of the nation's most prominent citizens, George Wythe of Virginia. Wythe was one of the Founders, a signer of the Declaration of Independence and a close friend of Thomas Jefferson. In 1806, while Jefferson was in the White House, Wythe was eighty years old and serving as high chancellor of the Virginia High Court of Chancery in Richmond. On May 25 of that year, he was taken violently ill after eating his breakfast, suffering stabbing pains in his stomach and chest and bouts of vomiting. Wythe's servant Lydia Broadnax, a free black woman, and his sixteen-year old protégé Michael Brown, another former slave, were stricken with the same symptoms.

When his physician arrived, Wythe claimed that he had been murdered. In spite of medical attention, his condition grew worse, and he died on June 8. Brown had passed away a week earlier. Of the three victims, only Lydia Broadnax survived. Although Wythe claimed that he had been poisoned, the three physicians who examined him gave the cause of death as cholera, a disease with symptoms similar to those of arsenic poisoning, even though there had not been a single recorded case of cholera in the United States up to the time.

Many people in Richmond, however, believed that Wythe had been poisoned, and their chief suspect was his grandnephew, George Wythe Sweeney, the black sheep of the family. Sweeney had free rein in the Wythe household, coming and going as he pleased. He was a compulsive gambler, and his granduncle had agreed to cover his debts on a number of occasions. He had also forged Wythe's name on checks several times and stolen rare books from his granduncle to sell for his debts. Recently, however, Wythe had told

Sweeney that he had had enough of the young man's antics and would cut him out of his will if there were any more thefts or forged checks.

Sweeney was arrested and indicted for the murders of Wythe and Brown. The evidence against him seemed strong. He had a financial motive for the murder of his granduncle, and Broadnax had seen him on the morning of the alleged poisoning, moving his hand over the top of the pot of coffee and then tossing a white piece of paper into the fire. He had poured his own coffee just before this point and then had left the house shortly thereafter. The investigation revealed further damaging evidence about Sweeney. A friend told the authorities that Sweeney had spoken to him about procuring some poison and that he informed Sweeney that it was easy enough to obtain ratsbane, a rat poison containing arsenic, at a store. Two slaves stated that they had seen Sweeney crush some white material into a powder with a hammer and then put it into a folded white piece of paper. The day after Sweeney was incarcerated, pieces of paper with white powder that appeared to be arsenic were found just a few feet from the jail wall, and the jailer suspected that Sweeney had thrown them over the wall during his exercise time. A similar white powder had also been found in Sweeney's room. To make matters worse, the brazen young man had forged his granduncle's signature on a check while Wythe was on his deathbed, which immediately aroused the suspicion of the teller, since everyone in town was aware of Wythe's grave illness. The bank president alerted the authorities, and Sweeney was arrested for forgery even before he was charged with murder.

Most residents of Richmond believed that Sweeney was guilty, and they assumed that there was no doubt that he would be convicted. But things did not turn out as expected. First, Virginia law prohibited blacks from testifying against whites in a criminal trial, so the testimony of Lydia Broadnax and the two slaves was not admissible. Even more damaging to the prosecution's case was that the three physicians who conducted the autopsies on the victims (the same ones who had treated Wythe during his fatal illness) would not state categorically that either Wythe or Brown had been poisoned with arsenic. They would only say that it was possible that one or both had been poisoned, but they stated that it was also possible they died as a result of gastrointestinal disease. Although there was no definitive test to detect arsenic in the body in 1806, there were various tests that the doctors could have performed, as in the case of Mary Blandy, that would have at least been suggestive. In addition, no effort appears to have been made to try to identify the suspicious white matter through any chemical tests. Even the anatomical examination of the two bodies was rather superficial. Perhaps not surprisingly in light of these developments, the jury took less than an hour to render a verdict of not guilty.

MADELEINE SMITH[20]

One of the best-known cases of arsenic poisoning is that involving the accusation against Madeleine Smith that she murdered her lover, Pierre Emile L'Angelier. Writers have continued to debate the case from the trial of Smith in 1857 up to the present, with no definitive consensus as to her guilt or innocence.

In the early morning hours of Monday, March 23, 1857, L'Angelier woke up his landlady, Ann Jenkins, by ringing the doorbell at the front door of her boarding house in Glasgow, Scotland. L'Angelier was violently ill and had to be helped to his room and his bed. He vomited a foul-smelling liquid. As L'Angelier's condition worsened, Jenkins fetched a doctor, who applied a mustard poultice and indicated that he would return later. In the meantime, L'Angelier asked Jenkins to send for his friend Mary Perry. By the time Perry arrived, however, it was too late. The doctor had returned before she got there and had pronounced L'Angelier dead.

L'Angelier's death was reported to his employer, the merchant firm W. B. Huggins and Company, and his direct supervisor, William Stevenson, went to the boarding house. Jenkins asked Stevenson to take responsibility for the belongings in L'Angelier's room. Among these items were a stack of letters from Madeleine Smith and a memorandum book. More letters from Smith were later found in L'Angelier's desk at Huggins and Company. The correspondence made it clear that Smith and L'Angelier had been carrying out a secret love affair for the past two years.

The two lovers first met in the spring of 1855, when Smith was nineteen and L'Angelier was thirty-one. He was from a French family that had settled on the British island of Jersey, in the English Channel. After spending some time as a young man in France and then in Edinburgh and Dundee, Scotland, he arrived in Glasgow in 1852, where he obtained his position as a clerk at Huggins and Company. But young L'Angelier apparently believed that he was destined for, and perhaps even deserved, a better position in life. Making a good marriage would be one easy way to achieve such a goal, and he had earlier pursued an unsuccessful relationship with a young woman from a prominent family in Fife. At some point in 1855 in Glasgow, he noticed Madeleine Smith. She was an attractive young woman who came from a prosperous Scottish family, which likely stimulated L'Angelier's interest in her.

It was not possible in Victorian society, however, for him to simply approach her and introduce himself. Given that she moved in much higher social circles than he did, the likelihood of their meeting at some social event was essentially nil. He did, however, finally get to meet her through a family member of a coworker who knew the Smith family. Madeleine seems to have been immediately taken by this handsome and charming young man. Thus began their acquaintance, which developed into a romance through secret correspondence and clandestine meetings. In June 1856 the relationship became a sexual one. Smith's letters to L'Angelier repeatedly refer to him as her husband.

But her family stood in the way of their union. Smith recognized that her family would never approve of a match with a poor clerk from an undistinguished family. Indeed, when her father learned that his daughters Madeleine and Bessie were seen on a number of occasions walking with a man unknown to him, he was furious and forbade Madeleine to see L'Angelier. Although Madeleine tried to explain her feelings to her parents, they would not hear of her marrying a mere warehouse clerk. She tried to break off the relationship several times, but she could not bring herself to do so, and L'Angelier refused to give up the hope of eventually marrying her. They made plans for a secret elopement that was postponed and never carried out.

The situation was further complicated in the middle of 1856 with the entrance onto the scene of William Minnoch, a bachelor in his early thirties and a senior staff member at a merchant and importing firm. Smith's father took a liking to Minnoch and began inviting him frequently to the family home. He obviously saw Minnoch as a good match for his daughter, and did what he could to promote such a union. As L'Angelier received reports of Smith frequently being seen in the company of Minnoch, he became increasingly jealous and upset. At some point, probably by late 1856, Smith's feelings toward L'Angelier began to change. Minnoch's attentions to her may have begun to have an effect, and she may have become tired of her clandestine

affair. She probably realized that Minnoch was going to propose to her soon
and that she would not defy her family's wishes by refusing him. The prospect
of living a life based on the salary of a clerk, with her family possibly cutting
her off from any support, may also have dampened her ardor for L'Angelier.
Her letters became somewhat cooler, but she still continued to profess to
love him and to want to marry him.

Smith must have felt increasing pressure to end her relationship with
L'Angelier. Finally, matters came to a head on January 28, 1857, when Minnoch
proposed marriage and Smith accepted. Now she was in a serious dilemma.
How was she going to tell the volatile L'Angelier that she was engaged to
another man? She saw an opportunity when L'Angelier, who was for some reason angry with her, returned one of her letters. She used this occasion as an
excuse to try to break off the relationship and asked him to return her letters.
He was despondent, but he refused to return the letters and instead threatened
to turn them over to her father. Smith wrote him again with a desperate plea
not to do anything until she could see him. She realized that she had to retrieve
these letters, which would spell an end to her marriage to Minnoch and shame
her and her family if they became known.

The matter of the letters remained unresolved until the time of L'Angelier's
death, when they were found among his possessions, as previously noted.
Perhaps suspicious because of the letters, his employer agreed to pay for a
postmortem examination. The appearance of the inner organs of the body
made the two autopsy doctors suspect the presence of a poison. The authorities were informed, and an investigation commenced. During the autopsy,
the stomach and its contents had been removed, and these were now sent for
analysis to Dr. Frederick Penny, the professor of chemistry at the Andersonian
University in Glasgow. Penny's analysis revealed the presence of one-fifth of
an ounce of white arsenic, which he indicated was "considerably more than
sufficient to destroy life." On the basis of the analysis and the letters,
Madeleine Smith was arrested on March 31 on the charge of murder.

Smith's trial began on June 30, 1857, in Edinburgh, as legal authorities had
decided that it would be best not to have the trial in Glasgow. The trial was
a sensation, with newspapers reporting on the case every day. It was
described as the trial of the century. The courthouse and the courtyard outside overflowed with reporters and curious onlookers as the proceedings

began. Smith was charged with two unsuccessful attempts to murder L'Angelier in February, as well as his murder in March. The two attempted murder charges were based on the fact that on these earlier occasions, L'Angelier had become violently ill with symptoms similar to those on the day he died, which doctors had determined were consistent with arsenic poisoning. Smith pleaded not guilty to all charges.

In addition to the initial examination of the contents of the victim's stomach, which had revealed the presence of a substantial quantity of arsenic, the prosecution brought forth further evidence of arsenic poisoning based on an autopsy performed after the body was exhumed. The famous Edinburgh toxicologist Robert Christison testified that he had analyzed nine portions of L'Angelier's body that had been sent to him and that he had found arsenic in all the samples. The question of what had killed L'Angelier was therefore clear, and even the defense did not dispute the fact that he had died of arsenic poisoning.

The prosecution argued that Smith had a strong motive to eliminate L'Angelier, who had threatened to turn her letters over to her father. The letters made it abundantly clear that the two had engaged in sexual relations and that they had considered themselves to be husband and wife. Passages from the letters were read in court. In addition, the prosecution was able to show that Smith had purchased arsenic on two recent occasions, signing the poison register and telling the pharmacist that the poison was for the purpose of getting rid of rats. She later claimed that she had actually brought the arsenic for cosmetic purposes, applying it to her face and arms after diluting it in water. Although the prosecution could not demonstrate that Smith had purchased poison in advance of the first alleged attempt on L'Angelier's life, she clearly had arsenic in her possession before the second alleged attempt and before his death. In addition, L'Angelier had apparently returned from a trip with the intention of meeting with Smith on the day of his death, although no evidence could be produced that the two had actually met on that date. According to the prosecution, he had gone to her house to talk to her that night, and she had administered poison to him, probably in a cup of cocoa, which she often served to him.

Of course, the defense challenged these claims. As to motive, the defense attorney argued that it was not in Smith's interest to murder L'Angelier while he was still in possession of the letters, as she must have realized that they might very well come to light upon his death. The arsenic she had purchased contained a small percentage of coloring matter, as required by law, but those who analyzed parts of L'Angelier's body made no reference to finding any coloring matter, although they testified that they had not been asked to look for it and had not done so. The defense also emphasized that there was no proof that L'Angelier and Smith had actually met on that fateful night. In response to the prosecution's argument that using arsenic as a cosmetic would be dangerous and did not seem reasonable, the defense had two pharmacists testify that other women had requested arsenic from them for this purpose. The defense also pointed out that the amount of arsenic found in the victim's stomach was very large and that presumably the amount he had taken would have been even larger, raising a question of whether or not such a large quantity of the chemical could have been satisfactorily dissolved in the cocoa and administered without his noticing anything wrong. The defense attorney provided evidence that in the past, L'Angelier had spoken to acquaintances about suicide, in connection with disappointed love affairs and suggested that he had taken the arsenic himself when he realized that his plan to marry Smith had failed. L'Angelier was painted by the defense as someone who wanted to move up in the world by marrying into a prominent and well-to-do family. Two defense witnesses also testified as to having heard him admit that he had taken arsenic at times for health or cosmetic reasons.

The case went to the jury on July 9. They took less than thirty minutes to render their verdict. On the first charge of attempted murder, Smith was found not guilty. On the second charge of attempted murder and the charge of murder, the jury rendered the peculiarly Scottish verdict of not proven. Under Scottish law, there is no real difference between not guilty and not proven, but the perception is that the latter verdict is used when the jury is not convinced of the innocence of the defendant but does not believe that the prosecution has made an adequate case against the defendant. It is sometimes jokingly stated that the verdict means, "We know you're guilty, but we can't prove it." Whatever the jury may have thought, the crowd in the courtroom and outside, which had been hostile to Smith at the start of the trial but had later taken her side, cheered wildly. Interest in the case continued even after the trial had ended, and the debate over Smith's guilt or innocence has continued up to the present time. Much has been written about the case, and it eventually became the subject of a feature film (*Madeleine*, directed by David Lean and released in 1949), as well as of episodes of two British television shows.[21] Smith's story was also used as the basis for other films, plays, and novels.

Did Smith kill L'Angelier, hoping naively that there would be no suspicion surrounding his death and that the letters would never be made public? Did L'Angelier, in a fit of disappointment, commit suicide? One recent book even makes the claim that he not only committed suicide but planned his death in such a way as to frame Madeleine for murder as a final act of revenge.[22]

FLORENCE MAYBRICK[23]

Another famous British murder trial of the nineteenth century involving arsenic poisoning was that of Florence Maybrick. Florence was born in 1862 in Mobile, Alabama, to William and Caroline Holbrook Chandler. Her father was a banker in the cotton trade. Her mother was a beautiful woman who attracted the attention of men, and there was gossip that she was having an affair with a Confederate officer. Early in 1863 William Chandler was stricken with a puzzling illness. His wife served as his nurse, and she refused admittance to his sick room to relatives who came to see him. When William died shortly thereafter, his family suspected that Caroline had poisoned him. If Mobile was not at the time being strangled by a Union blockade, it is likely that an investigation would have occurred. No action was taken, but Caroline, with public opinion against her, soon moved to Macon, Georgia, with her two children. There she married Capt. Franklin Bache Du Barry, the Confederate officer who had been her suspected paramour in Mobile.

In 1864 Du Barry and his new family sailed for Scotland. He died while onboard the ship. Caroline and her children continued on to Britain but after a brief time moved to Paris, where they spent the next few years. They returned to the United States after the Civil War had ended, but Caroline was back in Europe again a year or so later, where she married Baron Adolph von Roques in 1872. They lived in Germany and in Russia for the next few years, but the marriage did not work out. By 1879 the baron had abandoned the family. Caroline then began a life of traveling back and forth between

Europe and America, indulging in scandalous conduct and incurring large debts. Her children were raised largely in institutions and in the homes of relatives and friends.

At the age of eighteen, Florence met James Maybrick onboard the liner *Baltic* in 1880 while traveling from America to Europe with her mother and brother. Maybrick, who was born in Liverpool, England, was forty at the time. He owned a trading firm and made frequent trips to America to buy cotton. By the end of the voyage, James and Florence were engaged, and they were married in London on July 27, 1881. The couple spent the next three years in Norfolk, Virginia, where Maybrick had established his American headquarters, but they moved to Liverpool permanently in 1884.

In 1887 the marriage began to run into trouble. In that year, Florie, as Florence was generally called, discovered that her husband was maintaining a mistress. James had been involved with this woman long before his marriage and was still seeing her. In addition, James admitted to Florie at about that time that he was having financial problems and that they would have to reduce their living expenses. She was not good at handling money and sometimes spent extravagantly. She also gambled on horses. The debts began to pile up, and Florie concealed them from her husband for as long as she could. As tensions increased, Florie began to seek emotional support from other men. Eventually she began an affair with Alfred Brierley, a cotton broker who was a friend of her husband. The Maybricks apparently came to the brink of separation and divorce but then reconciled.

In late April 1889, James became ill and had a vomiting attack. By April 28 his illness had become serious enough to call a doctor, who diagnosed chronic dyspepsia and placed James on a diet. At the time, Florie expressed her concern to the doctor about a "white powder" that her husband, who was apparently a hypochondriac, was taking. Although James soon recovered, he fell ill again on May 3. His condition worsened over the following days, and Florie suggested to James's brother Edwin that perhaps they should call another doctor. Edwin asked William Carter, professor of materia medica and therapeutics at University College, Liverpool, to examine James on May 7. Carter initially reaffirmed the earlier diagnosis of dyspepsia, occasioned by ingesting some irritant food or drink. Michael Maybrick, another brother of James's, later told Dr. Carter that he suspected that his sister-in-law might possibly have been poisoning her husband. Michael had arranged for Florie to be relieved of James's care and had hired a nurse for this purpose. When the nurse reported that she had seen Florie remove a bottle of a meat extract prescribed for James from the sickroom and then later return it, Michael turned the bottle over to Dr. Carter for analysis. Carter found a "metallic irritant" in the meat juice and decided that further analysis was necessary.

When James died on May 11, there were enough suspicious circumstances surrounding his death that his brothers searched the house and found large quantities of arsenic in various places, as well as some incriminating love letters in Florie's room. Dr. Carter also refused to sign the death certificate. The police were informed of the situation and immediately placed Florie under house arrest while an investigation took place. The bottle of meat extract removed from the sickroom did contain arsenic, but James had never taken this preparation after Florie had it in her possession. The postmortem examination of James had not produced any definitive evidence of arsenic in his body. Michael, however, insisted that the body be exhumed and further testing be done. At this second autopsy, examiners found about one-tenth of a grain of arsenic in the kidneys, liver, and intestines. A coroner's jury ruled that Florie, who was by this time in jail, had murdered her husband, and she was committed for trial.

The trial began on July 31, 1889. There had been a huge growth in the number of British newspapers since the time of Madeleine Smith's trial, so the Maybrick case received even more press attention. Evidence against Florie included her affair with Alfred Brierley (which could have provided a motive) and her seemingly unhappy relationship with her husband; the fact that she had purchased flypaper containing arsenic during the time of James's illness; the observation by the Maybricks' nanny that she had seen the flypapers soaking in a basin of water (a method for extracting the arsenic) in Florie's room; and the nurse's testimony that Florie had removed from and later returned to the sickroom a bottle of meat extract, which was subsequently found to contain arsenic.

Her attorney, however, provided a strong defense. He pointed out that the amount of arsenic in James's body was very small and that it could have come from medicines that James was taking (although it should be noted that much of the arsenic in his body could have been eliminated before he died). He provided evidence that James did frequently use arsenic for health purposes (or possibly as an aphrodisiac) and that he was a hypochondriac who took various medications, including toxic ones such as strychnine. One local druggist testified that James came into his shop regularly for an arsenic "pick-me-up."

Florie had purchased the flypapers, the defense attorney argued, to prepare an arsenic water solution for cosmetic purposes (as Madeleine Smith had earlier claimed about her purchase of arsenic). As for the meat extract, Florie maintained in a written statement that she had removed it from the room to add to it, against her better judgment, some white powder that James had insisted she administer in his food. In attempting to explain why she had removed the bottle, Florie may have damaged her own case by admitting that she added a white powder to the meat extract. Although James did not drink from this bottle after Florie returned it to his room, her admission of this action probably did not help her in the eyes of the jury.

The trial, however, seemed to most observers to be going in Florie's favor. The press, which had initially assumed her guilt, had come around to believe in her innocence, as in the Smith case. In summing up the evidence, however, the judge gave a presentation that was clearly biased towards the prosecution's case. Possibly illustrating his disapproval of her infidelity, he practically asked the jury to deliver a guilty verdict, and after only thirty-eight minutes, they did just that. Florie was sentenced to death, creating a public outcry, including a petition signed by almost half a million people. The queen, on the advice of the home secretary, commuted Florie's sentence to life in prison.

In both Britain and the United States, Florie's supporters continued their efforts to obtain her freedom. One of the affidavits collected in this campaign was from one Valentine Blake, who swore that in January 1889 James Maybrick confided to him that he took arsenic whenever he could get it, thus confirming evidence given at the trial. According to Blake, James told him about Styrian peasants, who took arsenic regularly for their health and vigor. The efforts to free Florie eventually bore fruit, and she was released from prison on January 20, 1904. She returned to the United States, where she died in 1941.

As in the case of Madeleine Smith, the Maybrick case has received significant attention over the years. In addition to a number of accounts of the case,

Florie's story also served as the subject of a play entitled *The Poisoner* and may have served as an inspiration for Dorothy Sayers's mystery novel *Strong Poison*. Florie was also displayed in wax at Madame Tussauds in London. Some of those who have written about the case, such as Trevor Christie and Victoria Blake, lean toward the view that she was wrongfully convicted.[24] On the other hand, in his recent book on the history of poison, John Emsley devoted a chapter to the Maybrick case and detailed why he was convinced that Florie was guilty.[25]

FREDERICK SEDDON[26]

Frederick Seddon was an insurance agent who lived with his wife, Margaret, and five children in a large house in North London. Seemingly obsessed with making money, Seddon also operated a secondhand clothes store in his wife's name and speculated in real estate. At some point, he met a middle-aged woman named Eliza Barrow. She had received a comfortable inheritance in stock and property that supported her and her friend's young nephew, Ernest Grant, whom she had taken in. She was apparently a difficult tenant for any landlord, and she moved frequently. In 1910 she rented several unoccupied upper rooms in the Seddons' house.

Over time Barrow came to rely more and more on Seddon for advice concerning her investments. At some point she transferred about £1,600 in stock to him in exchange for a small weekly annuity and remission of her rent for the rest of her life. Apparently, Barrow's other investments also came under Seddon's control.

In early September 1911, Barrow began to suffer agonizing stomach pains, and a doctor was called in to see her. He prescribed bismuth and morphine. During Barrow's illness Seddon persuaded her to make a will leaving all that she possessed to Ernest Grant and his sister Hilda, with Seddon as the executor. Barrow's condition worsened over the coming days, and she died on September 14. The doctor who had attended her issued a death certificate without even examining the body, stating that her death was due to natural causes. Seddon quickly arranged for a cheap funeral, and Barrow was buried in a common grave, although her family had a burial vault that Seddon probably knew about.

Barrow's death benefited Seddon because he no longer had to make payments on the annuity or provide her with rent-free accommodations. On the surface, it appeared as if the chief beneficiaries of her death were the Grants. Of course, as the executor, Seddon had substantial control over whatever assets remained in her estate until the children were of age.

When Barrow's cousin, Ernest Vonderahe, came to call on her, he was shocked to learn from a servant that she had died about a week earlier and had already been buried. The Vonderahe family became suspicious about the sudden illness and death of their cousin and her quick burial. Over the next few weeks, Seddon spoke with several members of the family, but he was extremely brusque with them and did not satisfy their concerns. Eventually the family went to the police with their suspicions. Based on Barrow's hasty burial in a common grave, Seddon's involvement in her financial affairs, and the doctor's description of the symptoms of her illness, the authorities decided to exhume Barrow's body. Several of her organs were removed and sent off for examination. The examining chemist's report clearly showed that there was a large quantity of arsenic in the body. An inquest was held, and on December 4 Seddon was arrested for the murder of Eliza Barrow. About a month later the police also arrested his wife on suspicion that she was also involved in the crime.

The Seddons' trial began on March 4, 1912. Counting against the Seddons were their financial interest in Barrow's death; their opportunity to poison her, since they served as her caretakers during her illness (and no one else had access to her); their failure to inform her family of her death; her hasty burial in a common grave; the symptoms of her illness; and the arsenic in her body. The prosecution also provided evidence that the Seddons' daughter Maggie had purchased arsenical flypapers shortly before Barrow fell ill. The arsenic in these papers can easily be extracted by boiling them in water. As in essentially all poisoning cases, the evidence was circumstantial, as rarely is a poisoner observed in the act of committing the crime.

The defense challenged most of these points. As to the purchase of the flypaper, for example, defense attorney Marshall Hall questioned the identification of Maggie Seddon as the purchaser of the flypaper in question. This evidence was based solely on the testimony of Walter Thorley, the druggist who sold the paper. Hall pointed out, however, that when originally questioned by the police, Thorley said he did not think he could identify the girl who purchased the flypaper. Later the police took him to headquarters

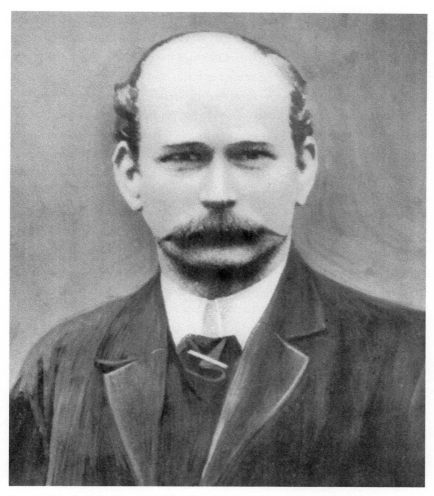

Poisoner Frederic Seddon. *From Filson Young, ed.,* Trial of the Seddons *(Edinburgh and London: William Hodge, 1914).*

and asked if he could identify the purchaser from a group of twenty people. He selected Maggie. Hall argued that Thorley would have known Maggie, since she had been in his shop on at least two other occasions and because she had been in his house twice as a friend of his daughter. In addition, Maggie's portrait had by this time appeared in the newspapers. Under the law, Thorley should have recorded the name of the person who purchased the flypapers, but he had failed to do so.

Interestingly enough, Margaret Seddon, in her defense testimony, also admitted to purchasing flypapers. She did so, she said, at the request of Barrow, who was bothered by the many flies in the room where she lay ill. This type of flypaper had to be placed in water, and Margaret stated that she placed four pieces of the paper in saucers in Barrow's room. She also testified that one day she accidentally broke one of the saucers containing the flypaper and that she then decided to transfer all four of the papers into one soup bowl with water and left the bowl on a table in the room. Hall suggested that perhaps the water from the bowl had accidentally been poured into something that was given to Barrow to eat or drink (possibly by the servant). This would explain the arsenic in the victim's body, and perhaps her death (although Hall maintained that it was also possible that she had died of epidemic diarrhea, which had similar symptoms to arsenic poisoning). Unfortunately for the defense, no one other than the Seddons (e.g., the servant, Ernest, the doctor) could remember seeing the flypapers in the sick room.

Hall tried to explain away other damaging evidence as well, but in the end the jury found Seddon guilty. It took them exactly one hour to reach their verdict. Margaret, however, was found not guilty. Frederick Seddon was sentenced to death and hanged on April 18, 1912.

HERBERT ROWSE ARMSTRONG[27]

Herbert Rowse Armstrong was a British lawyer who had served in the army and achieved the rank of major, a title he used for the rest of his life. The major joined a law practice in the little English town of Hay-on-Wye in 1906, and the following year he married Katherine Mary Friend, who by all accounts possessed a strong personality and dominated her husband and children. A teetotaler and opponent of tobacco, she would not let her husband drink and allowed him to smoke in only one room in the house. She often rebuked and humiliated him in public, as on one occasion when she dragged him away from a tennis match while loudly proclaiming that it was his bath night.

In 1920, Katherine, who was somewhat of a hypochondriac, underwent a decline in her mental health, suffering from delusions. Her doctor asked a colleague to examine her as well. The doctors found her to be listless, and they had difficulty getting her to speak. They concluded that she was of unsound mind and recommended to Armstrong that she be sent to Barnwood, a private asylum, for treatment. The major agreed. After a few months, her condition improved, and she asked her husband to obtain her release. When Armstrong made this request to the director of the asylum, the doctor argued that Katherine still suffered from depression and that he could not discharge her. The major insisted, however, and he removed her from Barnwood on January 22, 1921.

By February 10, however, Katherine was complaining of severe pains and vomiting, and her skin was discolored. Her doctor visited her the next day and gave her a thorough examination, but he could not reach a clear diagnosis. Her health continued to deteriorate, and in the early hours of February 22 the end seemed near. Her doctor visited her that morning and told the major that he did not think she would last for the rest of the day. Strangely enough, Armstrong said he had a lot of work to do and asked the doctor to give him a lift to his office. Katherine died shortly after the two men left the house. There was no suspicion of any foul play, and she was buried on February 25.

There the matter might have rested except for an incident later that year involving the sale of some property. The transaction had actually been initiated in late 1919, when the buyers paid a deposit of five hundred pounds to Armstrong, who was the lawyer for the seller. The sale was supposed to be complete by February 1920, but Armstrong kept finding reasons for putting it off. The buyers finally ran out of patience and instructed Oswald Martin, the lawyer who now represented them, to inform Armstrong that if the transaction was not completed on October 20, 1921, the contracts would be rescinded and the major would be asked to refund the deposit. The date came, and Armstrong claimed that he needed an additional week, but the buyers refused. On October 21 formal notice of the withdrawal of the contracts was sent to Armstrong's office. It was later revealed in the trial that Armstrong was having financial difficulties and was probably not in a position to refund the deposit at that time.

Martin was a competitor of Armstrong's in Hay, and relations between the two men were not exactly warm. Yet at this point Armstrong issued an invitation to Martin to come to his house for tea. Eventually Martin agreed, and the date was set for October 26. Armstrong served buttered scones and currant bread along with the tea. That night Martin became violently ill with vomiting and diarrhea. The doctor diagnosed a bilious attack, and Martin recovered. But Oswald's father-in-law, a pharmacist named John Fred Davies, became suspicious and spoke to the doctor, Thomas Ernest Hincks, who had also been Katherine Armstrong's doctor. Davies pointed out that the symptoms of a bilious attack were similar to those of arsenic poisoning, and he noted that he had sold Armstrong arsenic, supposedly as a weed killer, on several occasions. He also mentioned that he did not trust Armstrong.

Davies also discussed his suspicions with the Martins and warned them that if he was right, another attempt might be made on Martin's life. At that point, the Martins told Davies about a box of chocolates they had anonymously received earlier that month. A visitor who had eaten one of the chocolates had later become ill, but no one connected the two events at that time. Davies asked for the chocolates and found evidence of tampering. He then decided to obtain a urine sample from his son-in-law, and he and the doctor sent the sample and the chocolates to a laboratory in London for analysis.

When the analysis revealed arsenic in the urine and in two of the chocolates, the situation came to the attention of the Director of Public Prosecutions. Meanwhile, Armstrong had been repeatedly asking Martin to come to tea again, and Martin offered excuse after excuse to avoid the encounter. After a police investigation, the police arrested Armstrong on December 31, 1921, and charged him with the attempted murder of Oswald Martin. At the time of his address, three love letters from a woman named Marion and a packet containing white powder, which was later shown to be arsenic, were found in Armstrong's pockets.

On January 2, 1922, police court hearings began in Hay on the question of whether there was enough evidence against Armstrong to commit him for trial. These proceedings soon took a dramatic turn, for on the day that they began, Katherine's body was exhumed. During the police investigation of Martin's illness, several people expressed concern about the death of the major's wife. In particular, Hincks, in thinking back on the symptoms of her final illness, had now come to the conclusion that she might have been poisoned by arsenic. An autopsy was performed on Katherine's body, and samples were sent to London for expert examination. The results revealed the presence of arsenic in every organ and tissue examined. The liver alone contained two grains of arsenic, usually a fatal dose. A new charge of murder was thus added to the charge against Armstrong.

The evidence against the major was deemed sufficient to commit him for trial, which began on April 3, 1922. After the brief proceedings of a grand jury, which had to issue a formal indictment, the actual trial began. The case against Armstrong was strong. Medical evidence clearly established that Katherine had died of arsenic poisoning, although the evidence that Martin had been poisoned by arsenic was less definitive. The major had purchased considerable quantities of arsenic, which he claimed that he had used as a weed killer. Especially damaging was the packet of arsenic (containing enough poison for a fatal dose) found on the major at the time of his arrest. At the trial, Armstrong claimed that he had taken part of the arsenic that he purchased and divided it up into twenty individual packets. He stated that he used one packet per dandelion to kill the weeds, although he could not account for why he had used only nineteen of the packets and still had one in his pocket or why the remaining packet happened to contain enough poison to kill a human. His weak explanation probably did not impress the jury. Moreover, the facts did not support the defense's argument that perhaps Katherine had committed suicide.

The prosecution was also able to clearly show motive in the case of the murder of Katherine Armstrong. Letters and a memorandum book belonging to Armstrong showed that he was involved with other women, including during Katherine's stay in the asylum. Apparently, while free of the influence of his domineering wife, Armstrong was enjoying his freedom. Even more damaging was evidence that Armstrong had forged a new will for his wife, which changed the conditions of her original will in his favor. In the end, the jury took only forty-eight minutes to find Armstrong guilty, and he was hanged on May 31, 1922. After his death, Armstrong had the dubious distinction of having a wax effigy of him displayed in the Madame Tussauds Chamber of Horrors. His story was also the subject of a 1952 program on the BBC radio series *The Black Museum* and was the basis of a 1994 British television miniseries entitled *Dandelion Dead*.

Multiple Murders
THE CROYDON MYSTERY[28]
In 1929 the residents of the quiet and respectable London suburb of Croydon were shocked by the revelation that three members of a single family had

been fatally poisoned with arsenic in a period of just under a year. The family in question was that of Violet Sidney, a divorcee whose husband had left her for another woman many years earlier. She lived with her unmarried daughter Vera in a house in South Croydon. Violet's other daughter, Grace, lived with her husband, Edmund Duff, in a house a block away from her mother. Tom, Violet's son, and his wife, Margaret, lived just a few doors from the Duffs.

The family, which appeared to be close-knit, suffered the first of three tragic losses in April 1928. Edmund Duff returned from a fishing trip on April 26 feeling ill. His illness did not appear to be serious, but he suggested to his wife that she call their family physician, Robert Elwell, and ask him to come to the house. While waiting for the doctor, Edmund tried to have dinner, but he could not eat much. He did, however, consume a bottle of beer.

Elwell visited Edmund after dinner, but he did not find anything abnormal. He prescribed a light diet, aspirin, and quinine (because Edmund had suffered from malaria in the past). By the time the Duffs were ready to go to bed, Edmund felt much worse and had vomited. The next morning he was still vomiting and had diarrhea as well. He also complained about pain in his throat. Grace called Elwell, but he was out on rounds. His partner, Dr. John Binning, came instead, and he diagnosed colic caused by something Edmund had eaten. Edmund continued to deteriorate throughout the day, in spite of further visits by Binning and Elwell. Both doctors returned late that night in response to a frantic telephone call from Grace saying that her husband was having trouble breathing. But they could not save Edmund, who died shortly after 11 p.m. on April 27.

Elwell reported the death to the Croydon coroner, Dr. Henry Beecher Jackson, stating that in his opinion, death was due to ptomaine poisoning from something Edmund had eaten. He indicated, however, that he was not comfortable signing a death certificate without further examination, so the coroner arranged for an inquest. The postmortem examination revealed nothing unusual, and the inquest jury returned a verdict of death by natural causes.

The second tragedy suffered by the family occurred less than a year later, in February 1919. Vera Sidney had not been feeling well since the beginning of the year, but on February 11 her condition took a turn for the worse. That night at dinner, Vera had some soup. Normally she was the only person in the household to eat soup, but on that particular night the cook, Mrs. Noakes, had decided to have a small serving of half a cup. She gave what was left of the soup to the cat. Both Vera and Mrs. Noakes became violently ill, and the next morning the cook found that the cat had also been vomiting.

Vera was feeling a little better by February 13. Once again she had soup, this time with her lunch. Her aunt, who was visiting, had a few spoonfuls of the soup as well. Both women later became ill. The aunt eventually recovered, but Vera continued to deteriorate, and she died on February 15. The cause of death was considered to be gastrointestinal influenza, and no inquest was held.

Less than a month later, Vera's mother followed her to the grave. The death of her favorite child greatly affected Violet Sidney. Her surviving children feared for her health. One of the medicines that Elwell prescribed for her was a tonic called Metatone, which is still sold in the United Kingdom today. On March 5 Violet complained to her daughter Grace that her last dose of the tonic had tasted very strong and had gritty sediment in it. She soon suffered from violent bouts of vomiting and diarrhea, and she claimed that she had been poisoned by the medicine. Grace arranged for Binning to come to the house. Later he was joined by Elwell, who insisted that there was nothing in the tonic that could possibly have harmed Violet. As her condition deteriorated, a specialist was called in, but he could not reach a definite diagnosis. He suggested that Violet might be suffering from either a mineral poison, perhaps copper, or ptomaine poisoning from some food item. That night, Violet died.

Binning collected samples of the remaining food from the dead woman's last meal and also took the bottle of Metatone. Because they could not reach a definitive conclusion about the cause of Violet's death, neither Binning nor Elwell would issue a death certificate. The Croydon coroner thus ordered a postmortem examination. Samples of various organs from the deceased woman were sent to specialists to be examined for bacteriological evidence of food poisoning or signs of any chemical poison. The police also collected a number of bottles from Violet's house, as well as the bottle of tonic and the food samples that Binning had taken. Tests revealed the presence of arsenic in the medicine and in the organs removed from Violet's body.

Given this evidence of arsenic poisoning, the authorities decided to exhume the bodies of both Vera and Violet Sidney. Chemical analysis revealed the presence of arsenic in Vera's body and confirmed the earlier finding of arsenic in Violet's body. These results raised suspicions about the death of Edmund Duff, and his body was also exhumed. Once again, examiners found arsenic in samples taken of his organs and tissues. In the original postmortem examination of Edmund, arsenic poisoning had not been suspected as a cause of death, and the analyst had not thoroughly tested for it, consequently missing its presence.

Three separate inquests were held, one for each of the deaths. In each case, the coroner's jury ruled that death was due to poisoning by arsenic. Vera and Edmund, the juries concluded, were murdered by arsenic "willfully admitted by some person or persons unknown." With respect to Violet, the jury ruled that there was insufficient evidence to determine whether she committed suicide or was murdered.

In spite of the conclusion that at least two murders had been committed, no one was ever prosecuted in connection with these crimes. The prosecution did not believe it had sufficient evidence to convict anyone for the murders. The Croydon murders remain an unsolved case.

The two studies of the case on which this present account is based, however, have come to the conclusion that the murders were committed by Grace Duff. Grace of course had ready access to her husband, Edmund, and could easily have administered poison to him, for example, in his beer. There is evidence of marital discord between Grace and Edmund. Edmund's ineptitude in financial matters may have been one of the factors affecting their marriage. Poor investing by Edmund led to the loss of a five-thousand-pound inheritance that Grace had received from her father upon his death. There was also gossip that Grace was having an affair with Elwell. Certainly their friendship went beyond the bounds of discretion for that time.

Grace also had relatively free access to her sister and mother and was at their home frequently. She also benefited financially from both of their deaths. She would have had no trouble obtaining arsenic. Weed killer containing arsenic was found at the Duff home and also in an unlocked shed at the home of Tom Sidney.

Some of the facts above applied to Tom as well. He also benefited financially from the deaths of his mother and sister. But Tom was well off, and thus had less of a reason to commit murder for profit than his sister did. In addition, there is no plausible motive for Tom killing Edmund Duff, and he would not have had an easy opportunity for administering the poison to Edmund. Grace clearly seems to be the most likely candidate to be the murderer, but it is not probable that the case can be definitively resolved after all these years.

A TOXIC TOWN IN HUNGARY[29]

In June of 1929, the police in the small Hungarian village of Tiszakürt received two anonymous letters accusing two local married couples of murder. In one case, the couple was said to have poisoned the husband's father and uncle, and in the other case the supposed victims were the couple's son and daughter-in-law. The police opened an investigation into the possible murders, and the wives in both cases soon broke under questioning and confessed the crimes. Both women named a midwife from the neighboring village of Nagyrév, Zsuzsanna Fazekas, as the person who supplied the arsenic used in the murders.

The arrest of the two couples involved, however, was just the tip of the iceberg. As the police investigated these murders, they soon uncovered evidence of a host of similar cases of arsenic poisoning in the town and in neighboring ones going back as early as 1911. By September they had arrested thirty-five people, all but one of them women. And by the end of the year, they had opened more than fifty graves, exhumed the bodies, and performed autopsies. Over forty of the corpses contained lethal amounts of arsenic. The trials of the accused murderers stretched out over two years. When they were over, six women had been sentenced to death (although only two were actually executed), and twelve others received prison sentences. In the other cases, the prosecution was unable to prove the guilt of the defendants, which was not surprising since many of the alleged crimes had occurred years earlier.

The reasons why these women murdered so many family members (mostly husbands, children, or elderly parents) are complex and not completely understood. One of the probable factors was that the women were trapped in bad marriages (e.g., where they were abused by a drunken spouse and had no way of escaping their situation). Divorce was viewed as a disgrace, and the woman usually saw no alternative to remaining in the marriage. Eliminating a "problem" husband, especially one who was an alcoholic or abusive, must have seemed like an attractive solution. One woman who helped a friend poison her husband did so, she testified at trial, because the friend's husband was cruel and treated her badly.

In cases where a mother poisoned a child (sometimes a newborn infant), she believed that the family was too poor to feed another mouth. Infanticide was one means of limiting the size of the family. Sometimes an elderly parent or in-law was murdered to receive an inheritance or because the person had become too much of a burden. Added to the other hardships that a peasant woman often had to endure, taking care of a severely ill person might have been too much for her. In one case, a woman who was being physically abused by an alcoholic husband also had to take on the job of caring for her blind, bedridden mother-in-law and her elderly father-in-law, who could not control his bowels. The woman murdered her father-in-law with poison obtained from a neighbor. There were even cases of women murdering husbands who returned from the war with debilitating injuries.

Historian Belá Bodó has pointed out that during World War I, the women of the region became much more independent in the absence of their husbands and brothers. They had to assume many of the tasks that would normally have been carried out by men. The women developed a strong, separate culture, and it was within this culture that the women conspired to commit murder and cover up the crimes.

Arsenic could be readily obtained from local shops in powdered form as a poison for rats and mice. The more popular method of obtaining the poison, however, was to soak flypapers in water to extract the arsenic and then use the resulting solution as a poison. Sometimes one of the women who distributed the poison would instruct the would-be poisoner on how to obtain the arsenic (as in the instances of flypaper use), while in other cases the distributor would actually prepare the poisoned food or drink and bring it to the victim. Since these women often served as traditional healers, no one was suspicious if they brought food and drink to an ill neighbor. In these cases, some of the women accused of poisoning relatives claimed that they did not know the food or drink they served was poisoned. They stated that they thought the relative was being given something to help heal or calm the person, but in most cases they were probably aware that the victim was being poisoned. Apparently the women were under the misconception that arsenic could not be detected in the body, a view undoubtedly strengthened by the fact that the murders went undetected for so many years.

Much of the blame for the poisonings was placed on the midwife Fazekas, who seems to have been the chief distributor of the arsenic. The evidence at the trials, however, suggested that other women were equally as responsible. It was especially easy for defendants to claim that Fazekas was the guilty party, since she was not around to defend herself. When the poisonings were uncovered, the midwife committed suicide before the police could arrest her. One journalist covering the trials compared Fazekas to "a fatuous Eastern deity, perpetually devouring something with her bloody teeth . . . declaring the death penalty over the sick, the lame, the ones with 'loose morals.'"[30]

As discussed earlier, poisoning was often associated with women. At one of the trials, the prosecuting attorney claimed that most poisoners are women because it is in their nature to enjoy the suffering of others, adding, "Women are cowards, therefore they murder insidiously."[31] Bodó has correctly pointed out that poisoning cannot be tied to the abstract "nature of women," as many believed at the time, but he went on to note that poisoning was probably a more suitable method of murder for women than more violent methods, because they were generally smaller and less strong than their male victims.[32]

This fascinating story was the basis for the 2002 Hungarian film *Hukkle* (the Hungarian word denoting the sound of a hiccup), directed by György Pálfi. The filmmakers did not depict the murders directly but only hinted at them until the end of the picture, when the mystery is revealed in the singing of an old folk song. There is no dialogue in the film, which centers on an old man with hiccups who observes the daily life of the villagers. The film was set in the village of Ozora, rather than in the area where the murders actually took place. Recently, however, Nagyrév's mayor has decided to try to cash in on the town's notorious past. He has urged the townspeople to use the murders as a tourist draw and has tried to buy the house where Fazekas lived. He argued that many places have used negative aspects of their history to their advantage and asked why Nagyrév should not do the same. He noted, "We are famous for arsenic. Some tourists might be tempted to come." But some residents still see the poisonings as a shameful part of the town's history and have no wish to resurrect and highlight these events. Others are skeptical about the prospect of Nagyrév becoming a hot tourist destination on the basis of its criminal history.[33]

THE PHILADELPHIA POISON RING[34]

In the winter of 1938–1939, the city of Philadelphia was rocked by the exposure of a criminal conspiracy involving poisoning in the city's Italian immigrant community. The ring leaders were two Italian-American cousins, Paul and Herman Petrillo, and a Russian Jewish immigrant, Morris Bolber, better known as Louie the Rabbi. Although he was not actually a rabbi, Bolber taught Hebrew and considered himself to be a mystic with magical healing powers. Many of the superstitious Southern Italian immigrants of South Philadelphia came to him for cures and lucky charms.

Paul and Morris became friends and decided to form a kind of loose partnership. Paul, who owned a tailor shop, also fancied himself a practitioner of witchcraft and faith healing, the art of *la fattura* (the use of occult practices such as magic potions to cast spells). Paul and Bolber would refer clients to each other as appropriate, and the pair looked for other opportunities to make money.

Paul also speculated in shady life insurance practices. In his tailor shop, he came into contact with a number of life insurance agents who told him about a scheme to essentially use life insurance as a form of lottery. The idea was to take out a policy—with oneself as the beneficiary—on someone who was in poor health and a bad risk. The hope of course was that the insured would not live long. Many insurance policies could be written with no medical examination, as the companies made enough money to cover the risks. Paul began to accumulate such policies. Some were taken out by the individual's wife or children and then generally assigned to Paul, and others were taken out by Paul himself (claiming that he was a relative of the insured).

Paul's cousin Herman, who was involved in such criminal activities as counterfeiting and arson, suggested that Paul could increase his profits on the insurance policies if he would just send the insured "to California," a euphemism for killing the individuals involved. Paul was at first wary of taking such a risk. Instead, he hoped to rely on la fattura to speed up the deaths of the insured.

Finally, however, Paul became impatient enough in one case to employ a quicker and more certain method than magic. He had convinced a woman named Anna Arena to purchase a life insurance policy on her husband, Joseph, through one of his agent friends. When Bolber's sorcery did not result in Joseph's death, Paul called Herman and told him to send the man to California. Herman enlisted the aid of two men, one of whom was Anna's lover, to assist him in the task. The men picked up Joseph for a fishing trip on June 30, 1932. Once on the boat, they dumped him overboard, hitting him with an oar to knock him unconscious. When Anna collected the insurance check for Joseph's "accidental" death, she turned it over to Paul, who divided it among those involved in the plan. Anna was happy to be rid of her husband and free to pursue her romance with her lover unhindered.

Emboldened by this success, Paul and Bolber embarked on a larger scheme of murder to collect insurance money. Bolber soon suggested a simpler means of eliminating victims, namely arsenic. Herman and others also played a role as needed. Bolber supplied the arsenic, and Paul identified insurance "clients," in most cases through their wives. Many of the women were willing accomplices who wanted to be rid of their husbands and who knowingly administered the arsenic or made it possible for Paul or his associates to do so. Others may have been duped into believing that they were giving their husbands a love potion.

The plan worked smoothly for several years and multiple murders. The conspiracy began to unravel, however, in 1938. Herman had become friends with Ferdinand Alfonsi, who assisted Herman in distributing counterfeit money and fencing stolen merchandise. Alfonsi had a beautiful wife named Stella, who was unhappy in her marriage. Herman began an affair with Stella, and he apparently convinced her that they should get rid of her unwanted husband and at the same time make a profit by taking out a life insurance policy on him. In spite of his history of murder and theft, Herman was not comfortable with carrying out the actual killing of his friend. When George Myer, an ex-convict and owner of an upholstery cleaning business, approached Herman for a loan, Herman instead offered him either $600 or $2,500 in counterfeit dollars if he would murder Alfonsi. Herman suggested hitting Alfonsi over the head with a lead pipe and then throwing him down the stairs in his house to make it look like an accident. Myer did not really want to carry out the murder, but he strung Herman along in the hopes of getting an advance from him.

Meanwhile, Myer, who had previously served as an informant for the Treasury Department, knew that the feds would be interested in learning about Herman's counterfeiting and the proposed murder. He contacted the Secret Service branch office in Philadelphia and told his story. The Secret Service already suspected Herman of counterfeiting and bootlegging, and it saw an opportunity to use Myer to get to Herman. Agent Stanley Phillips was assigned to the case and went undercover as a hit man. Myer introduced him to Herman, explaining that Phillips was going to assist him in killing Alfonsi. The pair managed to stall Herman, finding one reason after another for delaying the job while they tried to obtain some counterfeit money from Herman. Eventually Herman agreed to sell them some counterfeit money.

Meanwhile, Herman grew tired of waiting for Myer and Phillips to murder Alfonsi, so he made other arrangements. He worked with Stella to poison her husband. When Myer learned what had happened, he informed the authorities. Alfonsi was seriously ill and was admitted to the hospital, where he died a month later. An autopsy revealed that his body contained large amounts of arsenic. Herman and Stella were charged with the murder of Alfonsi, and Herman also faced counterfeiting charges for selling counterfeit money to Phillips. Stella denied knowing anything about the murder, but eventually Herman, in an effort to save his own skin, began to reveal details about a number of murders. He claimed that he himself was innocent, but he identified his cousin Paul and Morris Bolber as the masterminds behind the poisoning ring. When Paul was arrested, he also claimed that he was innocent, and he placed the blame on Herman and Bolber. When Bolber was arrested, he also claimed innocence and provided information on others involved in the conspiracy.

The district attorney's office began to investigate various deaths based on information from the Petrillos and from insurance records. The large number of cases uncovered took the Philadelphia court system nearly a year to adjudicate. The Federal Bureau of Investigation (FBI) offered its laboratory facilities to assist the Philadelphia authorities in the examination of the many corpses that were exhumed. A total of twenty-five poison cases were prosecuted, with twenty-two convictions and three acquittals (including Stella Alfonsi). The women involved were dubbed "poison widows" by the press. At the conclusion of the trials, prosecutors attributed thirty-five deaths to the ring. They suspected, however, that the number may have been considerably higher. The Petrillos were both found guilty and sentenced to death. They were executed in the electric chair, Paul in 1940 and Herman in 1941. Bolber was also found guilty but somehow managed to escape with a life sentence.

Arsenic and Murder in Recent Years

All of the above examples of homicide involving the use of arsenic occurred in the period before World War II (with the Philadelphia murder trials concluding in the early years of that conflict). In more recent times, the use of arsenic as a poison in cases of murder has become less common but has by no means completely disappeared.[35]

There have even been two cases of arsenic poisoning in the twenty-first century. Eric Miller was a pediatric AIDS researcher at a cancer center at the University of North Carolina (UNC) Hospitals. His wife, Ann, worked at the pharmaceutical firm Glaxo Wellcome in Research Triangle Park.[36] On the night of November 16, 2000, Ann took Eric to Rex Hospital in Raleigh. He was complaining of severe stomach pains following a bowling outing the previous evening. Eric was admitted to the hospital, and by November 18 his condition had deteriorated to the point where they placed him in the Intensive Care Unit. That evening, one of the doctors at the hospital began to suspect arsenic poisoning as the cause of Eric's illness. He ordered a blood test, which revealed that there was a huge amount of arsenic in Eric's blood.

As Eric's condition worsened, he was transferred to the UNC Hospitals in Chapel Hill. He improved significantly and was discharged on November 24. But he became violently ill again on December 1 and was readmitted to Rex Hospital. By this time, a second set of tests done at UNC Hospitals while Eric was there had also revealed the presence of arsenic in his blood. Efforts to save Eric's life failed, and he died on December 2, 2000. The autopsy report concluded that Eric had died of chronic arsenic poisoning, which had taken place over a period of months. His death was the first recorded homicide by arsenic in North Carolina since a turkey farmer had been poisoned by his wife in 1997. It was only natural under the circumstances that Ann would be a suspect in the death of Eric, but there was insufficient evidence to indict anyone at the time.

The police investigation of the case continued for several years. One homicide detective in particular, Chris Morgan, doggedly pursued the investigation. Little by little he discovered that Ann was not the devoted wife that she appeared to be. Morgan uncovered evidence that Ann had engaged in several extramarital affairs. One of the men with whom she had been involved was a coworker named Derril Willard. He had been at the bowling alley with Eric the night before Eric was admitted to the hospital for the first time. The police learned that Willard had poured the beer for the men in the bowling group that night, and they speculated that he might have poisoned Eric's beer. Arsenic was readily available in the laboratory where Ann and Willard worked. When police questioned Willard, he indicated that he would not say anything until he had talked with his lawyer, Rick Gammon.

Willard was clearly very troubled by the police investigation, especially when news of his being a possible suspect appeared in a front page story in the *Raleigh News and Observer* on January 22, 2001. Shortly thereafter, presumably troubled by the consequences of his actions, Willard committed suicide. His death was a blow to Morgan, who had hoped to convince him to implicate Ann, whom Morgan believed had put Willard up to the attempted murder and had later administered the fatal dose of arsenic to Eric. It was possible that Willard had discussed his involvement in the case with Gammon, but client-attorney privileges prevented Gammon from revealing the content of their conversations without a court order.

The legal process wound all the way up to the North Carolina Supreme Court, and Gammon was eventually forced to turn over the information about Willard to the prosecution. The court order was narrowly written and stated that Gammon only had to provide any information that he might have about Ann's involvement in the murder, and not anything incriminating against Willard. Gammon revealed that Ann told Willard that while in the hospital room alone with Eric, she had injected the contents of a syringe into Eric's intravenous line. Although Gammon could not recall whether Willard had mentioned arsenic, he stated that Willard indicated that Ann had taken the substance in the syringe from work and that Willard knew the substance was poisonous. Although the date on which Ann carried out this action was not mentioned, Morgan suspected that it was during Eric's first hospital stay, when his condition, which had been improving, suddenly took a turn for the worse. Although Eric survived this particular attempt, the evidence was clearly damaging to Ann.

Ann Miller was arrested on the charge of murdering her husband, and the trial was set to begin in January 2006. The police and the prosecution were convinced that Ann would go to trial, but she surprised everyone by accepting a plea bargain, pleading guilty and receiving a sentence of a minimum of twenty-five years in prison. The case was finally closed.

An even more recent example of the use of arsenic for homicidal purposes involved the poisoning of members of the congregation of the Gustaf Adolph Lutheran Church in New Sweden, Maine, in 2003.[37] After a service at the church on April 27 of that year, parishioners gathered in the church hall to drink coffee and punch. Some of the churchgoers remarked that the coffee had a funny taste that day. Later that afternoon, a number of the coffee drinkers began to feel sick, with sixteen of them eventually becoming seriously ill. Laboratory tests revealed that the brewed coffee contained large quantities of arsenic. Prompt use of antidotes, particularly British anti-Lewisite (discussed in the next section), saved the lives of all but one of the victims, Walter Reid Morrill, whose death was ruled a homicide.

People in the small town of New Sweden were stunned by the news that someone had intentionally poisoned the coffee at the Lutheran church. They suffered a further shock a few days later when Daniel Bondeson, a longtime church member, was found at the family farm where he lived, with a gunshot wound to the chest. Bondeson was rushed to the hospital, but he died within days. Although police never had the opportunity to question Bondeson about the shooting, a note found near where he lay indicated that the death was a suicide. The note also served as an implied confession and began with the words, "I acted alone. I acted alone."

Most people who knew Daniel were shocked. He was known as a likable, decent person. Even though he had a college education, most did not think of him as being very bright. Some people thought that if he was involved in poisoning the coffee, someone else must have planned it and convinced him to do it. The police apparently also believed that Bondeson did not act alone, despite the opening words of his suicide note.

Suspicion fell upon Daniel's sister Norma, an outspoken woman disliked by many in the congregation. She had been actively involved in strenuous debates at the church involving such matters as whether the church should emphasize Swedish traditional values or take a new direction. The police continued to investigate the crime, with particular emphasis on Norma. In a detailed study of the case published in 2005, however, journalist Christine Ellen Young dismissed the theory that others (especially Norma) were involved in the poisonings. She argued that Daniel most likely acted alone, suggesting that he was mentally unstable. One individual she interviewed suggested that Daniel, who was also upset about the rift in the church, might have been angry about the way his sister was treated in the controversy. A source close to the Bondeson family told Young that Daniel might have been motivated by anger against people who he felt had created dissension in the church and whom he believed had mistreated and forced out the pastor. The source added: "Danny's perspective was that these people had taken over. He felt these others were in control, and improperly so. It was unethical. The church was his anchor too. When he killed himself, I think he was truly remorseful. The only thing that gave the conspiracy theory any drive is that the police were at a loss [as to] how to investigate it."[38]

New evidence came to light in 2006 with the testimony of Peter Kelley, an attorney whom Daniel Bondeson had consulted. Kelley had originally declined to discuss his conversation with Bondeson because of attorney-client privilege, but a court ruled that Bondeson's suicide note had waived the privilege. According to Kelley, Bondeson had visited him a few days after the poisoning incident and explained that he had put the arsenic in the coffee because he believed that someone at the church had once put chemicals in his coffee, which had given him a stomachache. Bondeson told Kelley that in order to retaliate, he poured liquid from an old spray can at the farm into the coffee, but he claimed that he did not know that it contained arsenic. Kelley said that Bondeson had not meant to kill or seriously injure anyone but just wanted to make them sick. With this information, the police officially closed the case, finally concluding that Bondeson had acted alone.[39]

The effects of the church poisonings were long lasting. Some victims continued to have health problems caused by the arsenic. In 2009 one of the victims died after a long battle with the effects of the poison. One can only imagine the social and psychological impact of the incident on the congregation and the broader community of New Sweden. The residents of the community, who largely wanted to put the poisonings behind them, were probably not thrilled by the story being featured in 2008 in a segment of the television show *Mystery ER* on the Discovery Health Channel.[40]

Arsenic and Chemical Warfare [41]

Chemical warfare is essentially a method of mass murder. While all warfare involves the murder of individuals, even when it is legally sanctioned, chemical warfare (along with biological and nuclear warfare) is considered to involve the use of a weapon of mass destruction. Most commonly, chemical weapons have been dispersed as gases. As early as 1899, a number of nations (not including the United States) signed the Hague Gas Declaration, which banned the use of projectiles whose sole purpose was the diffusion of asphyxiating or other deleterious gases. However, during World War I, every belligerent nation defied the ban on chemical weapons.

In an effort to break the stalemate of trench warfare, the Germans initiated the first large-scale use of chemical weapons in 1915, at first relying on chlorine gas, a lung irritant. The Allies quickly developed gas masks that were effective against chlorine, and the Germans introduced more toxic gases, such as phosgene. Eventually the Germans developed mustard gas, which had the advantage of being able to penetrate clothing and cause painful blisters and serious injury. The French and the British retaliated with their own mustard gas.

The United States, which did not enter the war until 1917, soon established a program to develop toxic gases and means of protecting against them. Originally under the Bureau of Mines, the program was transferred to the army in 1918 and became the Chemical Warfare Service (CWS). Chemist Winfred Lee Lewis, on leave from Northwestern University, headed one of the chemical warfare units at Catholic University of America (CUA) in Washington, D.C. Lewis was asked to develop a gas that would be even more effective than mustard gas, the effects of which were generally delayed and not typically fatal. It is perhaps not surprising that he and his staff began to experiment with arsenic compounds, given the long history of arsenic as a poison par excellence. Others on both sides of the conflict had earlier tried arsenic compounds but had not hit upon one that was an effective chemical warfare agent.

Lewis was approached by Father John Griffin, a chemist on the CUA faculty. Griffin remembered that he had had a graduate student, Julius Aloysius Nieuwland, who had completed a doctoral dissertation in 1904 on the chemical reactions of acetylene with various substances. One of the substances that he combined with acetylene was arsenic trichloride. The reaction produced a black, tarry mess that gave off a nauseating odor. He inhaled some of the fumes and became seriously ill, resulting in his being hospitalized for several days. It occurred to Griffin that whatever toxic compound Nieuwland had produced in this reaction might prove useful as a chemical warfare agent, and he showed Nieuwland's dissertation to Lewis, who decided to follow up this lead.

Lewis eventually succeeded by the use of distillation techniques in producing three poisonous arsenic compounds, one of which was deemed to be the most toxic and the best candidate for military use. This compound, dichloro(2-chlorovinyl)arsine came to be known as Lewisite. After purifying the chemical, Lewis and his colleagues tested it on animals and even on men. Much of the testing of the gas was done at the American University Experimental Station (AUES). Hundreds of stray dogs were gassed, as well as monkeys, goats, cats, rabbits, and other animals. Volunteers among the soldiers at the facility also underwent testing with Lewisite in several ways, such as having a very small amount of the chemical placed on the volunteer's arm. Occasional accidents at AUES involving pipes that leaked or vats that boiled over resulted in casualties and even fatalities.

There was one incident where a pipe attached to a still became obstructed, causing an explosion. Eight to ten pounds of Lewisite were released into the atmosphere, injuring some of the soldiers. A cloud of the gas drifted to the nearby home of retired senator Nathan Bay Scott, who was sitting on the back porch with his wife and sister. They felt intense pain in their eyes when exposed to the gas and promptly went into the house, where they closed all the windows and summoned help. Physicians from AUES arrived with respirators, and later the senator and his family received treatment from his physician. Fortunately, their injuries were not exceptionally serious, but the incident led to calls to move the testing from the American University site. The end of the war two weeks later, however, rendered the issue moot.

In the tests at AUES, Lewisite was found to be more toxic and more effective than mustard gas. The army began to produce large quantities of the chemical, which they expected to use in an Allied offensive planned for March 1919. Lewisite was never used in the war, however, because Germany unexpectedly surrendered in November 1918. Other arsenic compounds developed for possible use as chemical warfare agents during World War I included Adamsite (diphenylaminechloroarsine) and methyldick (methyl-dichloroarsine).

Lewisite was hailed as a major achievement of American science in the popular press after the war. Exaggerated accounts of its incredible toxic powers appeared in newspapers and magazines, and it became known as the dew of death. Lewisite was even featured as a poison used for criminal purposes in fictional works. In reality, however, the poison was not as effective as it was hyped to be. For one thing, Lewisite hydrolyzes (breaks down) when it comes into contact with water or water vapor. Apparently the Germans had developed the poison on their own before Lewis's work, but they rejected it in favor of mustard gas precisely because of this problem.

In the years following World War I, there was a debate concerning the ethics of chemical warfare. Some individuals (including, not surprisingly, many in the CWS) argued that it was actually a humane weapon when compared to the other instruments of death used in warfare. The general public, however, was repelled by the idea of chemical warfare, and even many in the military believed that the use of these weapons was dishonorable. In 1925 the League of Nations sponsored a conference at which participants approved the Geneva Protocol, which banned the use of chemical and biological weapons, although not outlawing their development or production. The protocol, however, contained no provisions for sanctions, verification, or enforcement. Many countries therefore continued to experiment with and stockpile chemical warfare agents.

When World War II began, a number of countries, fearful that their enemies would use chemical weapons in spite of the Geneva Protocol, rushed to try to find antidotes to poison gases such as mustard and Lewisite. The British were successful in developing an antidote for the latter, appropriately named British anti-Lewisite (BAL). Biochemist Rudolph Peters and his colleagues at Oxford University built upon the knowledge that arsenic attacks sulfhydryl (SH) groups in enzymes in the cells. They found that compounds containing two sulfhydryl groups (dithiols) exhibited great potential as possible antidotes for Lewisite. They synthesized and tested more than forty such compounds and found one that was extremely effective, namely BAL. Despite its success, it is still not clear whether BAL acts in the way proposed by Peters and his coworkers.

Although the nations of both the Allies and the Axis stockpiled chemical warfare weapons, including Lewisite, for possible use in World War II, these weapons played almost no role in the war. The Japanese army, however, did use mustard gas and Lewisite against the Chinese. Human experimentation with poison gases was also carried out by various nations during the war. Over four thousand American soldiers and sailors were intentionally exposed to high concentrations of mustard gas or Lewisite in secret World War II experiments. In 1993 the Department of Veterans Affairs agreed that the veterans involved could claim compensation for a list of medical problems that might have resulted from the tests.[42]

During the Cold War, some countries, particularly the United States and the Soviet Union, continued to experiment with and produce chemical warfare agents. Over time, most nations concluded that certain chemical agents, such as Lewisite, had become obsolete, and generally they disposed of their supplies by dumping them in the ocean. Eventually negotiations between many nations led to the Chemical Weapons Convention (CWC), which entered into force in 1997 and has been signed by over 180 countries. The CWC prohibits all chemical weapons and provided extensive and detailed verification procedures.

Lewisite and other chemical warfare agents have continued to create problems in some areas where these products were tested and manufactured. In the 1990s construction workers in the Spring Valley section of the District of Columbia began to uncover rusted bombs, shells, laboratory equipment, and other materials left over from the chemical warfare work carried out by the army at American University during World War I. Some of these materials tested positive for Lewisite and its degradation products. The army undertook remediation efforts and in 1995 claimed that all poison gas–related materials had been removed. The very next year, however, workers planting a tree on the grounds of the home of the president of American University were overcome by odors and suffered eye burns. Testing revealed high concentrations of arsenic in the soil. Further excavations by the army in the area eventually uncovered more shells, as well as drums and bottles containing chemicals such as mustard gas and Lewisite. The army began removing and replacing soil at properties in the neighborhood that had high levels of arsenic. Although some residents filed a civil suit against the army for alleged health problems associated with these chemicals, the court ruled that the government could not be held responsible because it appeared that the burial of these materials was not in violation of the army's policy at the time of World War I. There are other known and suspected sites contaminated with Lewisite in the United States, as well as in other countries, most notably Russia. The work of cleaning up these sites continues to this day.[43]

CHAPTER TWO

Poison in the Plot
Arsenic in Fiction

Given arsenic's popularity and notoriety as a poison in the history of civilization, it should not be surprising to learn that it has also frequently been employed in fiction. Arsenic has played an especially important role in detective or crime fiction, although it is also present in other genres, from pulp fiction to classic literature.

Arsenic in Detective Fiction

Arsenic is one of the most commonly used toxins in literary works, especially mysteries. Toxicologist John Harris Trestrail III has analyzed 187 works of detective fiction that involve criminal poisoning and compiled a list of the poisons employed and their frequency of use. Arsenic came out third on his list, appearing thirteen times, behind only cyanide (twenty-five) and mushrooms (fifteen). Of the seventy or so other poisons identified by Trestrail, none was employed more than six times.[1]

Although there were novels and stories that could be considered mysteries published before the nineteenth century, most scholars date the beginning of the detective story to Edgar Allen Poe's short story "The Murders in the Rue Morgue."[2] In this work, Poe introduced his brilliant French detective, C. Auguste Dupin, a private citizen who solves a murder that baffles the police (a common theme in detective fiction). Dupin also appeared in two later stories, "The Mystery of Marie Rogêt" (1842), based on a real-life murder, and "The Purloined Letter" (1844). In each case, Dupin uses amazing deductive powers to solve a crime, much like his later fictional colleague, Sherlock Holmes.

Many consider Wilkie Collins's *The Moonstone* (1868) to be the first detective novel,[3] although it was originally published in serial form (as were many of the novels of the time) in *All the Year Round*, the magazine of his friend Charles Dickens. T. S. Eliot called the book "the first, the longest and the best of the modern English detective novel." This was soon followed by the publication of six installments of Dickens's own mystery novel, *The Mystery of Edwin Drood*, in 1870. Dickens died before he could complete the work, but the unfinished novel was soon issued in book form.

The most famous detective in all of fiction appeared in the following decade, with the publication of the novel *A Study in Scarlet* in 1887. The detective was Sherlock Holmes, and the author was Sir Arthur Conan Doyle, a physician who enjoyed more success as a writer. Holmes uses superior intellect, astute observation, deductive reasoning, and forensic science to solve the most puzzling of mysteries. With the four novels and fifty-six short stories that feature Holmes, the genre of detective fiction was firmly established.

Poe did not make any use of poisons in his Dupin stories. In spite of his main character's forensic expertise, Doyle used poisons sparingly in the Holmes canon. Holmes's companion and the narrator of the stories, Dr. John Watson, noted that the great detective encountered only ten poison victims. None of these cases involved arsenic. The third of the early founders of detective fiction, Wilkie Collins, did utilize arsenic in one of his later novels, *The Law and the Lady*. Published in 1875, the book involves what may possibly be the first example of arsenic poisoning in a work of detective fiction.

The Law and the Lady revolves around the narrator, an English woman named Valeria Brinton, who in the first pages marries and becomes Mrs. Eustace Woodville, or so she believes. Valeria soon becomes aware that her husband's true surname is Macallan. When she confronts him with the question of why he married under a false name, Eustace refuses to discuss his past.

Undaunted by her husband's warning that if she learns the truth about this matter, their marriage will come to an end, Valeria decides to play detective in an effort to uncover Eustace's secret. She discovers that Eustace had been married previously and that his first wife, Sara, had died of arsenic poisoning. Worse still, Eustace had been tried for Sara's murder. The trial took place in Scotland, where the couple lived at the time, and resulted in a verdict of not proven. Eustace feels that because of this ambiguous verdict, he has

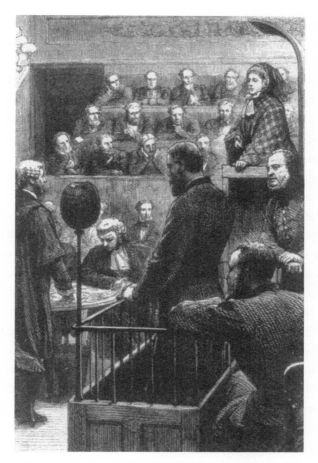

Frontispiece from Wilkie Collins, *The Law and the Lady*
(New York: Harper and Brothers, 1875).

not truly been declared to be innocent. He is dismayed that Valeria has
learned about the trial and believes, in spite of her protestations, that she
will never again be able to trust him or feel comfortable living with him.
Eustace leaves Valeria, but she, convinced of his innocence, is determined to
clear his name and win him back.

From the trial transcript, Valeria learns that Sara Macallan died at home
under suspicious circumstances. The doctors in attendance refused to sign
the death certificate and informed the police that Sara's symptoms were consistent with arsenic poisoning. A postmortem examination revealed that her

body contained enough arsenic to kill two people. There was sufficient circumstantial evidence against Eustace to charge him with the murder of his wife. His own diary revealed that he could barely stand his wife and that he had long been in love with another woman, who happened to be a guest in the Macallan home at the time of Sara's death. Two local druggists testified that Eustace had purchased arsenic, and the poison registers from the two pharmacies, which were signed by Eustace, confirmed their testimony. Eustace had also been observed serving his wife a cup of tea and administering her medicine on the day of her death. He thus had motive and opportunity to commit the crime.

The defense admitted that Eustace had purchased the arsenic, but he claimed that he bought it at the request of his wife, who said that the staff needed it to kill insects and mice. When these staff members were questioned, however, they denied ever having made such a request. Since his wife handled household affairs, Eustace said that he did not question her about it. He testified that he delivered the arsenic to his wife and never handled it again. The defense then argued that Sara actually wanted the arsenic to improve her poor complexion, a purpose that she did not want to reveal to her husband. To support this interpretation, the defense called upon two of Sara's friends as witnesses. They both testified that they had discussed with her the use of arsenic as a cosmetic, including mentioning the custom of arsenic eating among Styrian peasants to produce an appearance of plumpness and good health. One of the friends also indicated that she had obtained a copy of a book on the arsenic eaters for Sara, and the book was found in Sara's room.

Jenny Bourne Taylor, in her introduction to an edition of *The Law and the Lady*, pointed out that Collins, in writing this novel, may well have drawn upon the real-life 1857 case of Madeleine Smith. The verdict in the Smith case was also not proven, and there are several other similarities to the case of Eustace Macallan. Smith claimed that she purchased arsenic for cosmetic purposes, and the defense also referred to the practice of arsenic eating by Styrian peasants in her trial.[4]

Valeria, with the assistance of a few friends, eventually solves the mystery. She discovers that Sara had read Eustace's diary and learned that he was sorry he married her and was in love with another woman. In despair, she commits suicide by taking the arsenic she had asked her husband to buy. *The Law and the Lady* is thus a murder mystery without a murder.

Arsenic was employed as a murder weapon in numerous later detective novels and short stories. Fiction writers have utilized in their plots many of the features of arsenic poisoning that we have already seen in real-life crimes, such as the arsenic eaters and the medicinal and cosmetic uses of arsenic. In addition, the fact that arsenic is tasteless and thus easily administered in food or drink, and the similarity of the symptoms of arsenic poisoning to gastric disorders also play a role in some fiction. The cumulative effect of arsenic on the body, the ease of obtaining arsenic (e.g., in the form of rat and insect poison or weed killer), and the use of detection methods such as the Marsh test also appear in these works. I need to issue a "spoiler alert" here, warning lovers of mysteries that in discussing examples of the use of arsenic in detective fiction I will in some cases reveal the solutions to the crimes.

One relatively early use of arsenic in detective fiction occurs in the "The Moabite Cipher," a short story by British writer R. Austin Freeman published in 1909. The story features Austin's best-known creation, Dr. John Evelyn Thorndyke, a London physician and scientific detective (perhaps a combination of Holmes and Watson). The character appeared in eleven novels and forty-two short stories. In this particular case, arsenic is not used to murder anyone but rather acts as a ruse to deceive Thorndyke.

The story revolves around a mysterious message written in the Hebrew language in Moabite (primitive Semitic) characters. The message was found on the body of a man who was killed in an accident while under police observation as a possible anarchist. The police consult Thorndyke about the message, and he refers them to an expert at the British Museum to get the document translated. The translated message, however, makes no apparent sense. It appears to be written in some kind of code.

In the meantime, Thorndyke receives a visit from a man named Barton, who seeks his help in connection with a mysterious illness that has afflicted his brother. Barton fears that his brother's much younger wife may be poisoning him. He asks Thorndyke to analyze a sample of arrowroot that he has taken from his brother's breakfast, noting that his brother complained that the arrowroot had a gritty feel that morning. The medical detective suspects that the poison involved may be arsenic, and he subjects the sample to the Marsh test. The analysis shows that the sample contains very large quantities of arsenic. In fact, the amount of arsenic is so great that Thorndyke is skeptical about Barton's story. However, he agrees to go with Barton to visit his brother at Rexford, about an hour and a half from London.

When they arrive by train at Rexford, Barton leaves Thorndyke in order to make inquiries about the carriage that was supposed to meet them at the station. Still suspicious, Thorndyke watches Barton and sees him cross over to the other side of the tracks and board a train heading back to London. Thorndyke quickly boards this train as well, aware that it is the last train back to London that night. He suspects that Barton has used the story about the poisoning of his brother in order to lure him away from London. Since the newspapers had given the impression that the mysterious coded message was in Thorndyke's possession, he surmises that Barton may have wanted him out of London so that he could search his apartment.

Thorndyke alerts the police, and they catch Barton and his henchmen in the act of ransacking the doctor's apartment. The police recognize the men as well-known thieves. Thorndyke also believes that he has solved the mystery of the Moabite message, and he obtains the original document for further investigation. He realizes that the Hebrew language and Moabite characters were designed to mislead anyone who tried to learn the message's secret and did not contain the true meaning of the message. Thorndyke finds that if the document is wetted, an English-language message written in indelible Chinese ink appears. The message reveals the hiding place of the loot from a robbery. Although arsenic was not the murder weapon, the plot reflects the fact that arsenic was still frequently used in homicides at the time, and hence came readily to Thorndyke's mind when the possibility of poisoning was raised.[5]

Freeman did, however, use arsenic for murderous purposes in one of his later Thorndyke novels, *As a Thief in the Night* (1928). The first victim is Harold Monkhouse, a man who suffers from chronic illness, including gastritis. While his wife, Barbara, is away from home working on a campaign for women's emancipation, Harold dies. A doctor who had been called in as a consultant on the case shortly before Harold's death was troubled by the fact that he could find no obvious cause for the patient's condition, and he took some samples of blood and bodily secretions from the patient to be analyzed. Using Reinsch's test, the analyst found appreciable amounts of arsenic. An investigation revealed that a bottle of medicine in the bedroom of the deceased contained a substantial quantity of arsenic, suggesting that the poison had been administered in this way. The verdict of the inquest was that the "deceased died from the effects of arsenic, administered to him by some person or persons unknown, with the deliberate intention of causing his death."[6]

Thorndyke is not convinced that the poison was administered by mouth, because the amount of arsenic in the stomach was small. He has reasons to suspect Barbara of the murder but cannot at first determine how she might have given the poison to her husband since she was away from home for about two weeks preceding his death. By methods too detailed to discuss here, Thorndyke comes to the conclusion that the poisoning involved an ingenious mechanism. Barbara had melted down some candles and then remolded them with the addition of arsenic. She then placed these candles with the supply that her husband used regularly in his bedroom, and he was slowly poisoned by the release of toxic fumes over a period of time. Thorndyke also discovers that Barbara had committed another murder, which had until then gone undetected, by the same method some years earlier. When she realizes that her crimes have been discovered, Barbara commits suicide by injecting herself with an overdose of morphine.

As historian James Whorton has pointed out, arsenic was in fact used in the manufacture of some candles in the 19th century, although they were not designed with murder in mind. In the 1830s a new product known as composition candles came onto the market in Europe. They were introduced by French candle manufacturers, who found that adding white arsenic to the stearin used to produce their candles kept the product from becoming brittle and gave it a smoothness and sheen that customers preferred. It is not clear how many people became sick because of these candles, but when the public learned that they contained arsenic, demand evaporated. In the 1850s, however, a new kind of arsenic candle appeared, one that was colored green by the use of Scheele's green (copper arsenite). Arsenical pigments such as Scheele's green and Paris green were widely used to color a host of products in the nineteenth century.[7] By the time of Freeman's Thorndyke novel in the twentieth century, such candles were no longer available commercially.

Candles were also used as the mechanism of arsenic poisoning in Phoebe Atwood Taylor's aptly titled *Death Lights a Candle*, published in 1932 and set in Cape Cod. The first person to die in the novel is Adelbert Stires. The medical examiner finds arsenic in his vomit but is uncertain about how the poison was administered. Stires had been in perfect health when last seen at 10 p.m. the previous night, but he was found dead at 5:30 a.m. If the poison had been in his food, the medical examiner explained, the dose would have had to be very large for him to have died that quickly, but the amount of arsenic in the vomit was too small. In addition, no one else who had been at dinner with Stires had showed any symptoms of poisoning. The case is investigated by local sheriff Asey Mayo. The situation becomes more complicated when arsenic is found in the medicine of three of the guests in the house, although none of them have taken the poisonous preparations. At this point, Asey comments that it seems as if the entire household is "a pack of arsenic eaters." He then goes on to explain about the arsenic eaters of Styria and similar phenomena, claiming that it is possible to develop an immunity to arsenic by taking increasingly larger doses over time. Mayo believes that when Stires died of arsenic poisoning, the killer deliberately planted the poison in various places to confuse the investigation.

The solution to how Stires was poisoned is discovered accidentally when the killer attempts to murder Mayo and a friend. He deliberately plants a key to a locked room where it will be found, thus enticing Mayo and his friend to investigate. Once they enter the room, someone closes and locks the door behind them. The light in the room is not working, but by striking a match they discover a candle on a shelf. They light the candle to provide some illumination but eventually begin to feel sick. Mayo becomes suspicious because of the funny smell and peculiar flickering of the candle, and he snuffs it out, realizing that it may be poisoned. After his rescue, Mayo has the candle analyzed by the medical examiner, who finds that the wick had been dipped in Paris green, an arsenic preparation. When the candle burned, it gave off fumes of arsenious oxide and probably also arsine. The medical examiner explained that Paris green had formerly been used in wallpaper, which under certain conditions would release toxic gaseous arsenic compounds. Since Stires was known for leaving several candles burning while he slept, it seemed obvious that his death was caused by someone substituting the poisoned candles for his usual ones. Before the killer's identity comes to light, the arsenic candles claim another victim. In the end, however, Mayo catches the murderer.[8]

Legendary detective-story writer Dashiell Hammett made use of arsenic in his 1929 short story, "Fly Paper." In this work, a man and a woman plan to get rid of the lady's boyfriend by poisoning him with arsenic obtained by soaking flypaper. The woman attempted to build up an immunity by taking slowly increasing doses of it over time so that she could poison her boyfriend without suspicion by partaking of the same food that he did. She apparently tried to build her immunity too quickly, however, and died of chronic arsenic poisoning. The clue to solving the mystery is provided by a copy of Alexandre Dumas's novel *The Count of Monte Cristo* in which the flypaper was hidden. The book contained a description of how to build up immunity to a poison by taking increasing doses of it each day.[9]

Arsenic poisoning is prominently featured in a novel of one of the more well-known mystery writers, Erle Stanley Gardner. The book in question is *The Case of the Drowsy Mosquito* (1943), featuring Gardner's famous criminal lawyer/detective Perry Mason. The first reference to arsenic occurs when Jim Bradisson and his mother, after a dinner at the house of a friend, suffer from what appears to be food poisoning. The gastrointestinal symptoms involved suggest the possibility of arsenic, although it is unclear why others served from the same dishes of food did not become ill. When someone pointed out that the Bradissons were both great salt eaters and had poured copious amounts of it on their food, the contents of the salt shaker were analyzed and found to indeed contain arsenic. Both of the victims recovered. Later on in the novel, several guests are again the victims of arsenic poisoning after having tea at the same home, this time the arsenic having been placed in the sugar bowl. Among the victims are Perry Mason and his secretary, Della Street, although both recover thanks to an antidote provided by a nurse. The third victim, Banning Clarke, did not survive, but was shot to death shortly before he would have expired from what the autopsy showed was a fatal dose of arsenic, leading Mason to speculate about who would be judged guilty of the murder if the person administering the poison were not the same as the person who shot Clarke.

Yet, Bradisson and his mother had not been poisoned by arsenic. They had mimicked the symptoms of arsenic poisoning by taking ipecac, which produced copious vomiting, and had later doctored the salt shaker with arsenic, to divert suspicion from themselves when they later spiked the sugar bowl. Ironically, their real target did not partake of tea that day.[10]

Another example of the use of arsenic in a novel is Paul Doherty's *The Queen of the Night* (2006), set in imperial Rome. Curiously enough, arsenic is never specifically mentioned in the book, but in the author's note at the end of the novel, Doherty makes it clear that he has arsenic in mind in connection with two incidents in the work. In one of these, a character is murdered by "some slow-acting potion which would start like indigestion" that was slipped into his wine. In the author's note, Doherty states that there are "many types of arsenic and their effects vary" and that it was "quite probable" that this character was killed by arsenic. The other incident involves a Christian martyr whose body is uncovered in a remarkable state of preservation, although the evidence found along with her body suggests that she had died some ten years earlier. The Roman populace, which had converted to Christianity by the time in which the novel was set, believed that the body's state of preservation was a miracle and referred to it as the "sacred corpse." They believed that "God preserved her body as a sign of her sanctity." Doherty notes that "arsenic also has the power to slow down, or even halt, the process of decomposition" and quotes A. W. Blyth's 1920 book, *Poisons: Their Effects and Detection*, in support of this point.[11] Arsenic does indeed appear to slow decomposition and was used extensively in embalming, however, its use in embalming appears to date back only to the nineteenth century. It is possible, of course, that arsenic could have played a role in the preservation of bodies before this time if the individual in question had been poisoned with arsenic, or if the ground in which he or she was buried contained significant quantities of the element or its compounds.[12]

Terri Blackstock's novel *Shadow of a Doubt* (1998), set in Louisiana, also makes use of arsenic as a murder weapon. The book opens with detective Stan Shepard suffering from severe gastrointestinal distress in the middle of the night. His wife, Celia, calls 911, and Stan is rushed to the hospital, where he lapses into a coma. A medical examination reveals that Stan has been poisoned with arsenic. The police learn that Celia's first husband died of arsenic poisoning and that she was the primary suspect in the murder. Celia was brought to trial for that crime. In the courtroom, a policeman testified that the officer supervising the investigation had made a string of inflammatory remarks about Celia, including a comment that the wife is always guilty in such cases. It was obvious to the prosecution and the judge that the jury was angered by this testimony, which suggested that the supervising officer was out to get Celia, and they realized that the credibility of the investigation was undercut. Convinced that the prosecution would not be able to obtain a guilty verdict under these circumstances, the judge dismissed the charges. Celia was never actually acquitted, however, and once again became the chief suspect in the poisoning of her second husband.

The situation looked bad for Celia when a search of the Shepard home turned up a box of rat poison containing arsenic trioxide. To make matters worse, Celia violated a court order not to visit her husband in the hospital, where she was caught in his room and arsenic was found in his IV bag. In the end, however, it is revealed that Celia's brother David was responsible for the murder of her first husband and the attempt on Stan's life and that he had tried to frame her in both cases. David had long resented his sister because she was the favorite child, and he was seeking revenge. David's plot is discovered with the aid of Stan, who has recovered from the poisoning. David is about to murder Celia, who has also come to realize that he is the guilty party, when Stan arrives in the nick of time.[13]

Finally, Bertram Atkey's *Arsenic and Gold* (1939) features a man who builds up a tolerance to arsenic because he wishes to cross a "desert of arsenic" in order to reach a volcano that is rich in gold. In Sharyn McCrumb's *If I'd Killed Him When I Met Him* (1995), a woman is proved innocent of poisoning her husband when it is discovered that the arsenic that killed him was in the drinking water of a house he was renovating. The house was adjacent to a Civil War cemetery, and the arsenic from the embalming fluid used on the corpses had leached out into the groundwater. A man is murdered in Hailey Lind's *Arsenic and Old Paint* (2010) by the arsenical wallpaper in his room, and an artist survives an attempt on his life; the villain had mixed acid with an arsenic-based green pigment to release arsine gas. As we have seen in a number of other examples, fiction followed fact in that these authors made good use of historical facts about arsenic (e.g., the Styrian arsenic eaters, the use of arsenic in wallpaper and embalming fluid) in their works.[14]

Arsenic and Agatha

Agatha Christie, the author of sixty-six detective novels as well as numerous short stories and plays, is one of the most widely-read English-language writers of all time. The prolific mystery writer made far more use of poisons in her work than any of her colleagues in the genre. Michael C. Gerald, in *The Poisonous Pen of Agatha Christie*, reported that one or more victims were poisoned in over half of her novels.[15] Gerald also noted that arsenic appeared "as a poison, suspected poison, reference or joke in almost one-quarter of all Christie's novels!"[16]

Given Christie's background, it is perhaps not surprising that she made such extensive use of poisons in her fiction. Agatha Mary Clarissa Miller was born in Torquay, England, on September 15, 1890, and she married Archie Christie in 1914. During World War I she took courses in first aid and served as a nurse at the Red Cross Hospital in Torquay. Her first significant exposure to drugs and poisons came in 1916 when she passed the practical pharmacy exam of the Worshipful Society of Apothecaries of London and became a dispenser at the Red Cross Hospital.[17]

In her work dispensing medicines, Christie became knowledgeable about the chemistry and physiological actions of drugs. She was especially fascinated by the subject of poisons. In her first novel, *The Mysterious Affair at Styles* (1920), she chose poison as her murder weapon. Christie biographer Laura Thompson wrote in relation to the idea for this book, "It came from Agatha's dispensing work and could not have come to her otherwise, as it entirely depends upon a knowledge of poisons. In fact, it is impossible to reach the solution to Styles without this knowledge: the reader may guess right as to the culprit, but the guess cannot be proved without knowledge of the properties of strychnine and bromide."[18]

Christie used a wide variety of poisons in her work, generally with scientific accuracy. As Michael Gerald explained, "The use of poisons was Agatha Christie's hallmark. She used poisons to dispose of or attempt to dispose of more characters—by murder or suicide—than any other detective fiction writer."[19]

The Mysterious Affair at Styles involved the use of poison, in this case strychnine, to commit murder. This work also introduced one of her best-known detectives, Hercule Poirot. The first time that Christie used arsenic as a murder weapon was in a 1932 short story, "The Tuesday Night Club" (although she had made a passing reference to arsenic as a poison in a 1930 short story, "The Coming of Mr. Quin").

"The Tuesday Night Club" featured another of Christie's most famous detectives, Miss Jane Marple. The work was first published in Britain in 1932 in a collection of short stories called *The Thirteen Problems*, and appeared in the United States the following year under the title, *The Tuesday Club Murders*. The first six stories involve a group of six people, one of whom is Miss Marple, who form a club that meets on Tuesday nights to discuss and try to solve real-life mysteries. In "The Tuesday Night Club," Sir Henry Clithering, who had recently retired as Commissioner of Scotland Yard, presents the first case.

The story involved a woman who had died suddenly under suspicious circumstances, prompting a postmortem examination, which revealed that the cause of death was acute arsenic poisoning. Suspicion fell on her husband, who benefited from a life insurance policy on his wife and who was apparently having an affair with another woman. But no one could determine how the poison had been administered, since the husband, wife, and the wife's companion all ate the same meal the night of the murder. The husband also would not have had time to specifically poison his wife's dinner, since he returned from a trip just as dinner was being served. No one was arrested in connection with the case at that time.

As the club members listened to the details of the case, Miss Marple seized upon a number of seemingly trivial points. For example, Sir Henry mentioned that the police had discovered a blotter containing some words that had been transferred from a letter written by the husband. The words of the letter that could be read referred to the fact that the man was completely financially dependent on his wife during her lifetime, and he also made a mysterious reference to "hundred and thousands," which the police took to mean the amount that the husband would inherit upon his wife's death. In point of fact, his inheritance was substantially less than hundreds and thousands, and he was able to explain away the letter. Miss Marple, however, correctly deduced that "hundreds and thousands" was a reference to pink and white sugar decorations that were typically placed upon trifle, which had been served for dessert that night.

This interpretation might have seemed insignificant in itself, but Miss Marple pointed out that the arsenic could have been administered in these little decorations. Sir Henry had already noted in passing that the wife's companion did not eat the dessert because she was dieting, and the husband could easily have scraped the hundreds and thousands off of his dessert if he knew that they had been poisoned. Miss Marple then suggested that the reference to hundreds and thousands in the letter was part of instructions to someone on how to administer the poison. But if that were the case, who was the husband's accomplice? Miss Marple reasoned that the hundreds and thousands could easily have been doctored by the maid, who had seemed emotionally distraught when she was questioned by the police. As it turned out, Miss Marple was correct. The husband had gotten the maid pregnant and had promised her that he would get rid of his wife so that he could be with her. So he poisoned the decorations with arsenic and told the maid to serve them on the trifle. The husband later abandoned the maid and the child for another woman. Before the maid died (about a week before this first meeting of the Tuesday Night Club), she confessed all on her deathbed. The group was greatly surprised that a sweet, elderly lady like Miss Marple was able to solve the mystery.

Christie did not use arsenic as a murder weapon in a novel until the publication of *Easy to Kill* (the British title was *Murder is Easy*) in 1939. The killer is this book is a deranged woman who murders six people by various means. In the first, she puts arsenic in the victim's tea. As there was no reason to suspect foul play, the victim's death was initially attributed to gastritis. It was only after several other suspicious deaths had occurred that the facts came out.

Christie also employed arsenic in *What Mrs. McGillicuddy Saw!*, a Miss Marple mystery originally published in Britain in 1957 under the title *4.50 from Paddington*. In *They Came to Baghdad* (1951), one character becomes ill with violent gastroenteritis, and a colleague suspects that he may have been poisoned with Scheele's green. It is never definitely established, however, that this is a case of arsenic poisoning. Another character in the book is murdered by poison, but the substance involved is never identified.

Murder by arsenic also occurs in two Hercule Poirot short stories. In "The Lernean Hydra" (1939), a doctor whose wife has died of what is ruled a gastric disorder seeks Poirot's aid in squashing rumors circulating in the town that he has poisoned his wife. The rumors are fueled by the close relationship between the doctor and the woman who serves as his dispenser. Poirot deduces that the doctor's wife indeed had been poisoned with arsenic, but not by the doctor. The crime was committed by the victim's nurse, who herself was in love with the doctor and hoped that he would marry her after the death of his wife. In "The Cornish Mystery" (1951), a woman is killed with arsenic administered by the fiancée of her niece as a part of a scheme to ensure that the niece inherits the family wealth.

Christie also featured arsenic in another short story, "Accident" (1929, originally published under the title "The Uncrossed Path"). The sleuth in this case is a former police inspector named Evans who has retired to the country. Evans recognizes a neighbor, Mrs. Merrowdene, as the former Mrs. Anthony, a woman who was tried nine years earlier for the murder of her husband with arsenic. The fact that her husband was known to be in the habit of taking arsenic and the lack of definite proof led to her acquittal, but Evans was not completely convinced that she was innocent. Fearful that she might attempt to poison her current husband, Evans visits the Merrowdenes, where he is invited to take tea.

While her husband is out of the room, Mrs. Merrowdene pours bowls (in the Chinese manner) of tea for the three of them while commenting that her husband's habit of borrowing these bowls for his chemical experiments is going to result some day in someone being poisoned (which Evans believes is her method of making a poisoning seem accidental). Suspicious that Mrs. Merrowdene has poisoned her husband's tea, Evans presses her to drink from Mr. Merrowdene's bowl. When she instead pours the tea into a pot containing a plant, Evans warns her against the use of arsenic. Satisfied that he has prevented a murder, Evans drinks his own tea, only to discover that he is the one whose bowl was poisoned. As he lies there dying, she smiles and informs him that she had no intention of murdering Merrowdene, the man she truly loves. It is likely, however, that potassium cyanide was the poison in the tea, based on the rapidity and nature of the symptoms and the fact that Mrs. Merrowdene had specifically mentioned this poison as an example of a chemical that her husband had been using in these bowls just a few days earlier.

Poisoners were not always successful. In Christie's short story "S.O.S." (1933), a father attempts to use arsenic to murder a girl that the family took in as a foundling when he learns that she will inherit a fortune. He plans to pass his own daughter off as the foundling child in order to get control of the money. By chance, however, a stranded motorist is forced to spend the night at the family's home, and he discovers and foils the plot.

Christie also sometimes used arsenic in order to mislead investigators. In *Funerals are Fatal* (1953), which was originally published under the British title *After the Funeral*, a murderer poisons herself (though not with a fatal dose) with arsenic to throw off suspicion. But the intrepid Hercule Poirot solves the case. In *The Mirror Crack'd* (1962, published under the title *The Mirror Crack'd from Side to Side* in Britain), another murderer put arsenic in her coffee to make it seem as if someone were trying to kill her. She did not drink the coffee, however, complaining that it had a bitter taste. Her husband has a sample of the coffee analyzed, and it is shown to contain arsenic. Aware that arsenic has no taste, he comments that his wife may have been wrong about the bitter taste, but that she had the right instinct in rejecting the coffee. He is aware of his wife's crimes but is doing his best to cover them up. Miss Marple, however, is not deceived, and she discovers the truth. In yet another novel, *Third Girl* (1966), a woman takes small quantities of arsenic to make herself ill in an effort to implicate another character, but once again Poirot uncovers the plot.

Although arsenic was sometimes used by men for homicidal purposes in Christie's writings, a majority of those who employed the poison were women, perhaps reflective of the common view that poison was more of a woman's weapon. Arsenic also appeared in lesser roles in other Christie novels or stories, such as a suspected poison that was later disproved or as a subject of discussion. A number of Christie's novels or stories, including some involving arsenic, have been made into feature films or television programs.

Strong Poison

Another famous female mystery writer, Dorothy L. Sayers, used arsenic as a murder weapon in the novel *Strong Poison* (1930) and in a short story, "Suspicion." Sayers was born in Oxford, England, in 1893, the daughter of a clergyman. She studied modern languages and medieval literature at Oxford University and began writing mystery novels in the early 1920s. Her first novel, *Whose Body?*, was published in 1923 and introduced her famous detective, Lord Peter Wimsey.[20]

Sayers first used arsenic as a murder weapon in her 1930 novel *Strong Poison*, which starred Wimsey and also marked the first appearance of Sayers's other primary character, detective novelist Harriet Vane.

The story opens with the trial of Vane for the murder of her former lover, Philip Boyes, who has died of arsenic poisoning. After the couple had been living together for about a year, they quarreled, and Vane walked out on Boyes, but he did not accept the break and repeatedly pressed her to marry him. The trial results in a hung jury because one juror, Miss Climpson (a friend of Wimsey's), refuses to vote for a conviction in spite of the strong case against the accused.

The autopsy suggested that Boyes had received a large and fatal dose of arsenic, first becoming ill and then dying three days later. That night Boyes had taken dinner at the home of his cousin, Norman Urquhart, and then visited Vane, where he again tried to persuade her to marry him, without success. Boyes had coffee while at Vane's house, and he became ill shortly after leaving her. It appeared likely that the poison had been consumed either at the dinner or in the coffee. It did not seem possible that Boyes could have been poisoned at dinner, so the prosecution argued that Vane had put the arsenic in Boyes's coffee. This view was bolstered by the fact that she had recently purchased arsenic and other poisons. Vane did not deny that she had made these purchases but claimed that she did so as part of the research for a detective novel that she was writing. In fact, at the trial her publisher produced a copy of the manuscript showing that the subject of the book was murder by arsenic.

The title of Vane's book, incidentally, is *Death in the Pot*. The phrase is from the Bible (King James Version, 2 Kings 4:38–41), where it occurs in the story of Elisha purifying a pot of stew. There was a famine in the land, and Elisha prepares a stew for the sons of the prophets from wild vines and gourds gathered in the field. As the men began eating the stew, they cried out "Man of God, there is death in the pot!" and could not eat the meal. Elisha put some flour into the pot, and the stew was no longer harmful. The English chemist Fredrick Accum, who published *A Treatise on Adulteration of Food, and Culinary Poisons* in 1820, used this quotation (with an image of a skull) on the title page of the book, and in his preface attacking the practice of food adulteration, stated: "It should tend to impress on the mind of the Public the magnitude of an evil, which, in many cases, prevails to an extent so alarming, that we may exclaim, with the sons of the Prophet, 'There is death in the pot.'"[21]

Wimsey attends the trial and is captivated by the defendant, and convinced of her innocence. As a result of the inability of the jury to reach a verdict, the judge orders a new trial, which is set to begin in about a month, and Wimsey sets out to try to find evidence to support Vane's innocence before she is tried again. Eventually, Wimsey's suspicions come to focus on the murdered man's cousin, Urquhart. Through surreptitious means, Wimsey learns that Boyes was named as the principal beneficiary in the will of an elderly, wealthy aunt, but that his death leaves Urquhart as the sole beneficiary.

Wimsey also acquires evidence, once again by methods that go outside of the law, of arsenic in Urquhart's possession. The problem is, however, that Wimsey cannot find any way that Urquhart could have administered the poison to Boyes. It does not seem possible that Boyes could have been poisoned at the dinner with Urquhart. Both men partook of every course, and the portions were served from common dishes by servants who were present throughout the meal and consumed the leftovers afterward. The only dish not served by the staff was a dessert omelet prepared by Boyes himself at the table and shared by both men. Urquhart did not partake of the wine that Boyes drank, but it was poured from a new bottle that was opened at the table, and the remnants were consumed by the servants. Yet Wimsey is convinced that somehow, the arsenic was administered at dinner.

Wimsey pores over all the relevant literature that he can get his hands on, including the published trial records of persons accused of arsenic poisoning, such as Florence Maybrick and Madeleine Smith, as well as books on forensic medicine and toxicology. Finally the solution comes to him. Urquhart must be an arsenic eater! He could have developed an immunity to arsenic by taking increasing doses over a long period of time. As he explains when he confronts Urquhart:

> Yes, well, about this arsenic. As you know, it's not good for people in a
> general way, but there are some people—those tiresome peasants in

Styria one hears so much about—who are supposed to eat it for fun. It improves their wind, so they say, and clears their complexions and makes their hair sleek, and they give it to their horses. . . . Anyhow, it's well known that some people do take it and manage to put away large dollops after a bit of practice—enough to kill any ordinary person.[22]

Wimsey reveals that the arsenic must have been present in the omelet, since this was the only dish where there was nothing left over for the servants to consume. He notes that a servant recalled that one of the eggs for the omelet was cracked and that Urquhart himself decided that it should be used in the omelet. Wimsey deduces that Urquhart could easily have introduced arsenic into the cracked egg earlier. By asking Boyes to prepare the omelet, he further diverted suspicion from himself. Finally, he did not drink anything at the meal so as to further reduce the likelihood of any poisonous effects of the arsenic on himself.

Wimsey obtains hair and fingernail samples from Urquhart that indicate that he has been taking arsenic for a long time. In spite of all of this circumstantial evidence and speculation, however, Wimsey has no direct proof that Urquhart committed the murder, so he tricks him into confessing the crime, thus saving Vane. After the murderer is arrested, Wimsey recites the line "Mithridates, he died old" from A. E. Housman's poem "Terence, this is stupid stuff" from *A Shropshire Lad* (1896), remarking that he doubts that it will apply to Urquhart. The poem was one of the works Wimsey consulted as he pondered over how the arsenic was administered. The reference is to the ancient legend of King Mithridates, who supposedly made himself immune to poisons as a protective measure by consuming small doses of various poisons every day. Housman writes:

> *They put arsenic in his meat*
> *And stared aghast to see him eat;*
> *They poured strychnine in his cup*
> *And shook to see him drink it up...*
> *I tell the tale that I heard told.*
> *Mithridates, he died old.*[23]

Sayers also used arsenic in an attempted murder in the short story "Suspicion" (1940). In this tale, Mr. Mummery begins to suffer gastric distress at the same time that news stories are circulating about a woman named Mrs. Andrews, whom the police are seeking for questioning in connection with a case of arsenic poisoning. Mrs. Andrews had served as a cook for a couple who were poisoned with arsenic—the husband fatally—and she disappeared after the incident. As it happens, the Mummerys had hired a new cook at about this time. The woman, Mrs. Sutton, claimed that she had been looking after her widowed mother for quite some time and hence could not provide any references. As the Mummery's previous cook had departed rather suddenly, they were anxious to get a new cook quickly and hired Mrs. Sutton in spite of her lack of references.

Mr. Mummery continued to suffer from gastrointestinal troubles, and began to get suspicious of his new cook. Could she possibly be the poisoner whom the police are seeking? He became even more concerned when he discovered that someone had been removing arsenical weed killer, the very poison employed by Mrs. Andrews, from the can in the potting shed. Then one night he came home late and found a note from Mrs. Sutton telling him that there was a cup of cocoa waiting for him in the kitchen that just needed to be heated. When he sipped the cocoa, he thought that it had a faint and unpleasant metal tang, so he spit it out. He poured some of the cocoa into an empty, washed medicine bottle and took it to his friend, a local pharmacist, for analysis. Using the Marsh test, the pharmacist found that the cocoa contained a heavy dose of arsenic (about five grains), which is why, he claimed, Mummery was able to taste it. In point of fact, however, even five grains of arsenic would not have any taste. Although a metallic taste in the mouth is one of the symptoms of arsenic poisoning, a sip of the cocoa, which Mr. Mummery spit out, should not have produced any immediate metal taste. Given the demonstration of Sayers's knowledge of arsenic in *Strong Poison*, it is likely that she was aware of this fact, but presumably her need for a plot device to allow Mr. Mummery to discover the arsenic in his cocoa led her to take a certain poetic license.

Leaving the pharmacist to inform the police, Mr. Mummery rushed home, fearful for his wife's safety. Just as he was about to tell Mrs. Mummery about the arsenic, the cook appeared and informed the Mummerys that the police had just captured Mrs. Andrews, the poisoner, in another town. Mr. Mummery realized that he had been mistaken about the cook. But of course there had been the large dose of arsenic in the cocoa. Who could have put it there? The story ends with the following words: "He glanced around at his wife, and in her eyes he saw something that he had never seen before. . . . "[24]

Arsenic in Other Literature

Although arsenic, not surprisingly, appears most frequently in detective fiction, it is also found in other types of literature. As in crime fiction, arsenic is most often mentioned in other genres in connection with poisoning, whether accidental or (more often) intentional.

One of the earliest, if not the first, mentions of arsenic in a literary work is in Geoffrey Chaucer's *The Canterbury Tales* (which dates from the late fourteenth century). In "The Canon's Yeoman's Tale," the Yeoman is critical of the Canon's alchemical experiments. In listing some of the chemicals that the Canon has employed, the Yeoman includes "arsenyk" and elsewhere mentions the arsenic sulfides "orpyment" (orpiment) and "resalgar" (realgar), but he does not provide details of their use.[25] Arsenic may also have been mentioned in passing in Ben Jonson's play *The Alchemist* (1610), although there is some question about this matter because of the terminology involved. H. C. Hart, the editor of a 1903 edition of the play, interpreted the word "Zernich" in the text to mean arsenic based on his claim that the name "Zerichum" was given to arsenic by several chemical writers, but this argument does not sound convincing.[26]

Arsenic began to appear with more frequency in literary works in the nineteenth century, which historian James Whorton has called "the arsenic century" because of the ubiquitous use of arsenic in crime, medicine, and industry. Whorton gives several examples of literary works involving poisoning attributed to the arsenic used to color wallpaper green. In an 1862 short story published in *Chambers's Journal of Popular Literature, Science, and Arts*, Frederick Staunton is the orphaned ward of an uncle who wishes to eliminate him in order to inherit his estate. The uncle sends young Staunton to live with a vicar, instructing the cleric to give Frederick the best room in the house, one that is covered with emerald wallpaper. Although the vicar is aware of a local legend that claims the house is haunted and that several deaths have occurred in the green room, he feels obligated to follow the uncle's instructions. Staunton becomes gravely ill but is saved when a renowned physician is called in and immediately recognizes that the young man is suffering from arsenic poisoning caused by the wallpaper. As soon as he is moved to another room he recovers, thus foiling his uncle's plot.

Within the next fifteen years, two novels involving arsenic poisoning by wallpaper had appeared in Britain. The first of these, appropriately titled *The Green of the Period; Or, the Unsuspected Foe in the Englishman's Home*, was published anonymously in 1869. This dull novel is basically a series of lectures to two friends about the dangers of green wallpaper by a man who had nearly died while living in a room covered in such paper. His goal is to rid England of "the green of the period." The second novel, *Minsterborough* (1876), was written by a London physician named Humphrey Sandwith. In this three-volume work, a man accused of poisoning his wife with arsenic is saved from a death sentence by the town's pharmacist, who shows that the green wallpaper in the lady's bedroom was laden with arsenic.[27]

At least one modern scholar has suggested that arsenic wallpaper might have been responsible for or contributed to the illness of the narrator in Charlotte Perkins Gilman's classic short story "The Yellow Wallpaper." Beth Sutton-Ramspeck's argument on this point might have been more convincing if the story had been entitled "The Green Wallpaper," but of course there could have been some green arsenical pigment in yellow wallpaper. In the story, a woman possibly suffering from postpartum depression is confined to a room for a "rest cure." Over time, she slowly goes mad and becomes convinced that there is a woman, or perhaps a number of women, trapped behind the wallpaper, and that she herself is confined in this way. She tears off as much of the wallpaper as she can, telling her husband at the end of the story that she has escaped and that he cannot put her back because she has pulled off most of the paper. Sutton-Ramspeck tries to relate some of the woman's symptoms to arsenic poisoning, although she admits that few of the typical symptoms of arsenic poisoning are present in the narrator of Gilman's story.[28] There have been numerous attempts to interpret the story, with most critics focusing on the psychological and symbolic aspects of the wallpaper, rather than on any kind of physical poisoning.[29]

Title page of novel *The Green of the Period*
(London: Routledge and Sons, 1869).

Undoubtedly the most famous novel of the nineteenth century in which arsenic played a role was Gustave Flaubert's *Madame Bovary*. The work was first published in serialized form in the French periodical *Revue de Paris* between October and December of 1856. While the story is tame by today's standards, the work was controversial at the time, and Flaubert was prosecuted for obscenity. The prosecution argued that *Madame Bovary* was an affront to public morals and blasphemed against the church. Not only was the protagonist an adulteress, but she clearly enjoyed her liaisons with other men. The defense pointed out the flaws in Madame Bovary's character and the bad end to which she came, arguing that the story thus reinforced moral values. In the end, Flaubert was acquitted. The work was published in book form in April 1857 and has been hailed as one of the great novels of all time. There have been several film and television adaptations of the novel.[30]

In the book, Dr. Charles Bovary, a medical practitioner in provincial northern France, marries Emma Rouault, the daughter of one of his patients. Emma is a beautiful young woman who has been educated in a convent. The popular novels that she has read, however, have instilled in her a desire for romance and luxury, neither of which the kind but shy and unambitious Charles is able to provide. Emma becomes bored with her married life, and she winds up having affairs with two men. She also runs up large debts by purchasing luxury items that she cannot afford. When her debts are called in and Emma cannot raise the money to pay them off, she commits suicide by taking arsenic. A heartbroken Charles, who loses all his possessions due to the debts, dies not long afterward, and the Bovarys' young daughter is sent to live with distant relatives.

Monsieur Homais, a neighbor of the Bovarys', is the town pharmacist and the source of the arsenic. One day Emma is present when Homais scolds his young apprentice for going into the locked depository (a small room where the pharmacist kept his utensils and merchandise) to get a pan, emphasizing that the room contains dangerous products. He cites a blue glass bottle containing white powder, which he reveals is arsenic. When Emma decides to commit suicide, she badgers the apprentice into taking her into the depository to get some arsenic that she claims she wants to use for killing rats. As soon as they get into the room, Emma seizes the blue bottle and draws out a handful of arsenic, which she immediately eats, warning the young man not to tell anyone about this incident, or the blame would fall on the pharmacist.

Emma goes home and writes a note to Charles that she instructs him to read the next day. But soon the symptoms of arsenic poisoning begin. Emma apparently has no knowledge of arsenic poisoning and thought she would simply go to sleep and die. Of course, that was not to be the case. She senses an acrid taste in her mouth, becomes extremely thirsty, and eventually begins to vomit profusely, causing Charles great concern. Flaubert describes her agony in detail:

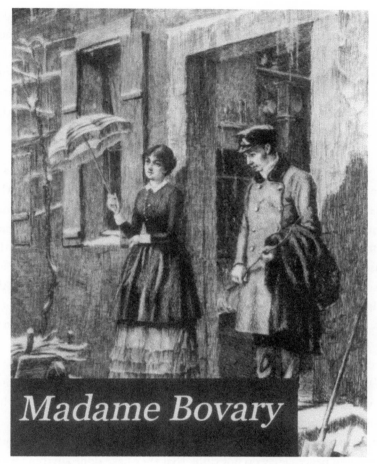

Cover of Gustave Flaubert's novel *Madame Bovary* (Paris: A. Quantin, 1885).

Beads of sweat were oozing from her bluish face, which looked as though it had been hardened in some sort of metallic vapor. Her teeth were chattering, her wide-open eyes stared vaguely around her, and to all his questions she replied only with a nod; she even smiled two or three times. Little by little, her groans became louder. A muffled scream escaped from her; she claimed that she was feeling better and that she would get up in a little while. But she was seized with convulsions, and she cried out, "Oh, God! It's horrible."[31]

A panicky Charles presses Emma to tell him what she has eaten, and she refers him to the note. He reads the message and repeatedly cries "Poisoned! Poisoned!" The maid runs to get Homais, and Charles explains the situation, begging the pharmacist to do something to save Emma. Homais, although mentioning an antidote, does nothing but talk about the need to do an analysis. Two other doctors are called in, but they conclude that there is nothing that can be done to save Emma at this point. Finally, with one last convulsion, she dies.

Even more so than *Madame Bovary*, the literary work most closely associated with arsenic is Joseph Kesselring's 1941 play *Arsenic and Old Lace*, which was made into a film starring Cary Grant in 1944. The story revolves around Abby and Martha Brewster, two elderly sisters who occupy a Victorian home in Brooklyn. The Brewster sisters have a habit of renting a room in their house to elderly men with no friends or family whom they then proceed to poison out of "kindness," helping these lonely men find peace, as Abby explains it. In spite of the title of the play, arsenic is actually only one of the poisons that the sisters employ. Not taking any chances that the poison will not do its job, the Brewsters concoct their deadly potion by adding arsenic, strychnine, and "just a pinch of cyanide" to elderberry wine.[32]

One day their nephew Mortimer finds the body of their latest victim in the window seat. When he confronts his aunts with this discovery, he is shocked to hear them calmly explain to him that this was only the latest of about a dozen men (all of whom are buried in the basement) whom they had helped find peace. They do not think that they have done anything wrong. Chaos ensues as poor Mortimer tries to stop his aunts from continuing their murderous ways while also doing his best to see that their crimes are not discovered.

Kesselring based his play on a true crime, the case of Amy Archer-Gilligan. Amy operated what was essentially a precursor of today's nursing homes in Windsor, Connecticut, in the early twentieth century. Elderly boarders paid either a lump sum for a guaranteed lifetime of lodging and care or a weekly rate for the same services. Amy preferred the lump-sum advance payment so that she had the boarder's money in hand. When the house became too crowded, Amy would free up a room and a bed by dispatching one of her clients with a dose of arsenic. This situation went on for years while Amy earned her living and kept her business afloat via the art of murder. Eventually her deeds were discovered, and Amy was arrested, accused of running what the press called a murder factory. She was charged with five murders, but authorities suspected that she was responsible for a much larger percentage of the sixty-six deaths that occurred in her home over a period of about nine years. Amy escaped the gallows by pleading guilty to second-degree murder in 1917, and she was sentenced to life in prison instead. While in prison, she either became mentally ill or faked such a condition, and she was transferred to a mental hospital, where she remained for the rest of her life. Unlike the fictional Brewster sisters, however, Amy did not commit her crimes out of "kindness," but for profit.[33]

A lesser known comic play that involves a murder plot utilizing arsenic is Charles Busch's *Die, Mommy, Die!* (1999), which was made into a film in 2003. The play is set in the 1960s and centers on Angela Arden, a middle-aged, former pop singer who is trapped in a loveless marriage with film producer Sol Sussman. Aware of her affair with a younger man, Sol cuts off Angela's credit cards and threatens to make her life miserable. She decides that it is time to get rid of him by putting arsenic in some warm milk that she offers him. Sol refuses to take the warm milk, complaining that he is constipated and needs to use a suppository. Angela quickly offers to assist him and, while he is not looking, dips the suppository into the poisoned milk. She assists Sol by inserting the suppository, surely one of the more novel methods of poisoning someone.

Actually, it turns out that Sol was not poisoned after all. He learned of Angela's plot to murder him from Bootsie, their maid, who discovered the arsenic in Angela's possession. In trouble with the mob because he could not pay back a loan, Sol decided that he would fake his death with the aid of Bootsie and some professional actors whom he hired to play police and medical personnel. Sol and Bootsie replaced the arsenic in Angela's vial with baking soda and proceed to carry out the plot. It is also revealed that Angela is actually her twin sister, Barbara, who murdered Angela and took her place years ago.[34]

If Flaubert is perhaps the most critically acclaimed writer to use arsenic in a novel, then his counterpart with respect to a short story is probably William Faulkner. Poisoning by arsenic plays a prominent role in Faulkner's

1930 short story "A Rose for Emily." Miss Emily Grierson is an elderly single woman who lives a reclusive life in an old decaying house, assisted only by her African American manservant. Years earlier, when she was in her thirties, the townspeople thought that Miss Emily would marry the foreman of a construction crew working on new sidewalks in the town. She was seen, for example, regularly riding with him in a buggy every Sunday afternoon, and she purchased a men's silver toilet set with the foreman's initials on it. But the foreman eventually disappeared, and nothing further was heard of him.

At about that time, Emily purchased some arsenic in the local drugstore. When the pharmacist informed her that she had to give a reason for her purchase of the poison, Miss Emily just stared at him and said nothing. Finally the pharmacist provided the arsenic, labeling the box "for rats." It was also about that time that Miss Emily's neighbors complained about a terrible odor coming from her house, but the smell went away after a week or two.

When Miss Emily died as an old, gray-haired woman, her house was inspected. On the bed in one of the rooms, they found the skeleton of a long-dead man. Upon the dressing table was a silver monogrammed toilet set, and the man's suit hung over a chair. Faulkner ends the story with the following words:

> The body had apparently once lain in the attitude of an embrace, but now the long sleep that outlasts love, that conquers even the grimace of love, had cuckolded him. What was left of him, rotted beneath what was left of the nightshirt, had become inextricable from the bed in which he lay; and upon him and upon the pillow beside him lay that even coating of the patient and biding dust.
>
> Then we noticed that in the second pillow was the indentation of a head. One of us lifted something from it, and leaning forward, that faint and invisible dust dry and acrid in the nostrils, we saw a long strand of iron-gray hair.[35]

Shirley Jackson also utilized arsenic poisoning in one of her works. Her 1962 novel *We Have Always Lived in the Castle* (which was adapted into a play in 1966) tells the story of the Blackwood family and is narrated by eighteen-year-old Mary Katherine "Merricat" Blackwood. Six years earlier, both Blackwood parents, an aunt, and a younger brother were all poisoned with arsenic mixed into the family sugar and sprinkled on blackberries. An uncle, Julian, was poisoned but survived and is confined to a wheelchair and is slightly demented at the time that the novel takes place. Merricat had avoided this fate because she had been sent to bed without dinner for misbehaving. Suspicion fell on her sister Constance because she did not put any sugar on her berries, and she was arrested and tried for the crime but eventually acquitted. The townspeople, however, are convinced that she is guilty, and the surviving Blackwoods become isolated from the rest of the community.

The story reaches its climax when Charles, a long-absent cousin, arrives at the Blackwood home. He befriends Constance, but his real purpose is to try to find the Blackwood fortune, which is locked in a safe in the house. Charles does not get along, however, with either Merrricat or Uncle Julian. When Merricat pushes Charles's lit pipe into a trash basket, a fire engulfs the house, destroying much of the upper portion. Julian dies in the fire, presumably due to a heart attack, and Charles is unsuccessful in his efforts to remove the safe. The two sisters flee to the woods for safety, and Constance informs her sister for the first time that she has always known that it was Merricat who had poisoned the family. Merricat put the arsenic in the sugar bowl because she knew Constance did not take sugar. The women return to what is left of their home to live out their lives.[36]

There are several examples of arsenic poisoning in recent literature. In Robert Goolrick's novel *A Reliable Wife* (2009), a mail-order bride in early twentieth-century Wisconsin plans to kill her new husband with arsenic. The wife, with the encouragement of her lover, begins to poison her husband slowly with small doses of arsenic. Goolrick writes: "It was everywhere. Arsenic. Inheritance powder, the old people called it. It was in his food, his water, on his clothing. It was on his hairbrush when he brushed his hair in the morning. He tasted it on the back of his tongue and in his throat. Not all the time, not every day, but always there. At first, the effect was tonic. He felt marvelous and strong. His skin looked ruddy and clear."[37]

But of course his health soon begins to deteriorate. Although he comes to realize that his wife is poisoning him, he decides to accept his fate. The wife, however, has pangs of conscience and decides she cannot go through with the murder. In the end, the lover dies, and the married couple is reconciled. The wife's pregnancy at the end of the story seems to suggest a new beginning.

Mary E. Lyons's novel for young readers, *The Poison Place* (1997) is based on real-life events. It tells the story of the Peale family of Philadelphia, centering on the father, Charles Willson, and two of his sons, Rembrandt and Raphaelle, all of whom were talented painters. Charles was also a devoted naturalist and established a natural history museum in 1786.[38] At the time, arsenic was widely used in taxidermy to preserve specimens. *The Poison Place* is narrated by Moses Williams, who was for many years a slave (later freed) of the Peale family and played an important role in the operation of the museum. The story tells of the friendship that developed between Moses and Raphaelle. In the book, Williams describes the deterioration of the health of Raphaelle, who did most of the taxidermy work. Raphaelle must certainly have known that arsenic was poisonous but continued to work with it anyway. He eventually died in 1825 at age fifty-one, possibly from years of exposure to arsenic, perhaps coupled with heavy drinking. In her author's note, Lyons writes: "Art historians agree that Raphaelle probably died of arsenic poisoning. They disagree about the reason. One suggests that Charles Willson Peale willfully allowed Raphaelle to use arsenic so that he could avoid it himself. Another says Peale was not aware that Raphaelle was sick from arsenic because heavy drinking disguised his symptoms. Some think Raphaelle knew arsenic was harmful, but performed taxidermy to please his father."[39] Raphaelle's death is discussed later in this book.

Arsenic was and still is used for various purposes in medicine, including alternative medicine. Arsenic is a remedy, for example, in the system of homeopathy and is mentioned in this connection in a recent short story by Niamh Russell. In "The Benefits of Arsenic" (2008), a woman offers two homeopathic arsenic tablets to a friend because arsenic "soothes your membranes." The skeptical friend takes the tablets, but thinks to herself, "I didn't even bother to ask her what were membranes or why mine needed soothing. Arsenic! What next? Cyanide for my stomach's sake? Strychnine for my stretch marks?"[40]

CHAPTER THREE

Hazards on the Job
Arsenic in the Workplace

Given the toxicity of arsenic, it is not surprising that individuals who have had to work with the chemical have often suffered negative effects on their health. The toxic action of arsenic on workers undoubtedly goes back to at least the Bronze Age. As Jerome Nriagu has shown, arsenic minerals tend to occur together with copper minerals in many places, and the primitive furnaces used in the smelting of these minerals would have generated copious fumes of toxic arsenious oxide. Exposure to these fumes would likely have adversely affected the health, and even threatened the lives, of smiths. Nriagu even suggests that the physical deformities typically shown in the depictions of the gods associated with fire and smiths, such as the Greek Hephaestus and the Roman Vulcan, may reflect occupational diseases linked to exposure to fumes of arsenic and lead. He concludes that "arsenic poisoning appears to have been among the first occupational diseases to afflict humankind."[1]

Arsenic in Mining and Smelting

Although little attention was given to occupational medicine in antiquity, the ancients were aware that certain diseases are associated with particular trades. The famous Greek physician Galen (second century AD) mentions some of the hazards faced by miners. He personally visited copper sulfate mines on Cyprus and noted that he was almost overwhelmed by the fumes. A number of ancient writers commented on the pallor of miners, which was probably due at least in part to poor ventilation. Measures were taken, some of questionable efficacy, to protect miners. Pliny the Elder (first century AD)

mentions, for example, the use of animal bladder skins as primitive respirators to reduce the inhalation of dust.

Mining in Europe declined dramatically during the Middle Ages, and
there is no further mention in the literature of occupational diseases associated with it until the sixteenth century, when the mining trade began to
expand. The classic description of the mining industry at this time is *De Re
Metallica* (1556), authored by the German Georg Bauer, who was better
known by his Latin name, Georgius Agricola. He was a physician who studied
the mining industry, and his book deals with all aspects of mining, smelting,
and refining, including the health hazards to the workers. Of particular interest is his mention of the poisons released by the fires that were set to break
the rocks in the mine. The fire produced fumes that led to nervous disturbances and loss of motor power among the workers. Medical historian
George Rosen, author of a book on the history of miners' diseases, suggests
that these workers suffered from arsenic poisoning. Arsenic was undoubtedly
a common component of minerals in the mines with which Agricola was
familiar.

The first book devoted specifically to the occupational diseases of miners
and smelters was by the unorthodox Swiss physician Paracelsus. Although
possibly written as early as the 1530s, it was not published until 1567, eleven
years after Agricola's book. Paracelsus clearly recognized and described
arsenic poisoning as one of the occupational hazards of miners and smelters.
He drew a distinction between acute and chronic poisoning, emphasizing
that ingesting the poison by mouth generally led to rapid sudden death, while
inhaling the fumes leads to a slower form of poisoning. Paracelsus discussed
the poisonous vapors that were given off when ores are roasted. Rosen has
pointed out that Paracelsus gave an excellent description of chronic arsenic
poisoning, "with the characteristic symptoms, pallor, thirst, gastro-intestinal
disturbances, and skin eruptions."[2]

Most historians consider Bernardino Ramazzini's *De Morbis Artificium
Diatriba* ("Of Diseases of Tradesmen"), published in 1700, to be the first
broad treatise on occupational medicine. Ramazzini was an Italian physician
who practiced and taught medicine in the city of Modena. In his book, he
describes how he first became interested in occupational diseases.

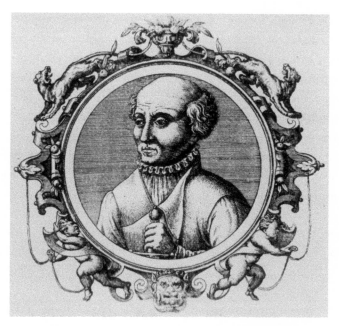

Paracelsus, who gave the first clear description of arsenic poisoning in miners. *Courtesy of the National Library of Medicine.*

In this city . . . it is usual to have the Houses of Office [privies or out-houses] cleaned every third year: and while the men employed in this work were cleaning that at my house, I took notice of one of them that worked with a great deal of anxiety and eagerness, and being moved with compassion, asked the poor fellow why he did not work more calmly and avoid overtiring himself with too much straining. This said, the poor wretch lifted up his eyes from the dismal vault, and replied that none but those who have tried it could imagine the trouble of staying above four hours in that place, it being equally troubling with the striking of one blind. After he came out of the place, I took a narrow view of his eyes, and found them very red and dim: upon which I asked him if they had any remedy for the disorder. He replied their only way was to run immediately home, and confine themselves for a day to a dark room, and wash their eyes now and then with warm water, by which means they used to find their pain somewhat assuaged.[3]

Ramazzini later discovered several beggars previously employed in this work who were now blind or nearly so. He then began to study the diseases associated with other trades, eventually leading to the publication of his book. In this work, he discussed the diseases of a wide variety of occupations, including miners, potters, surgeons, pharmacists, painters, blacksmiths, masons, and corpse bearers.

Ramazzini specifically mentions arsenic poisoning in connection with two occupations, "metal-diggers" (miners) and "chymists" (pharmacists). In his discussion of the unhealthy air present in mines, he cites the toxic fumes in arsenic mines and mentions the use of glass masks to protect workers from these fumes. With respect to pharmacists, he discusses the hazards involved in the preparation of certain medicines; arsenic compounds were used extensively in medicine over the ages. Ramazzini mentions a man who became seriously ill during the process of subliming arsenic when he breathed in some of the fumes.[4]

Arsenic poisoning was also mentioned by authors writing on the occupational diseases of miners in the eighteenth and nineteenth centuries, such as C. L. Scheffler and Phillipe Patissier.[5] Physicians who investigated these problems generally recognized that arsenic tended to produce a chronic form of poisoning in miners and smelters exposed to it. For example, the important British pioneer in occupational medicine, Charles Turner Thackrah, wrote in his influential 1832 treatise on occupational health, "The mines which contain arsenic are very baneful to the operatives, though the diseases which they induce are of slow march." He cited slight fever, colic, and weakness of the limbs as symptoms of chronic arsenic poisoning.[6]

Although exposure to arsenic frequently occurred in connection with the mining and smelting of other minerals such as copper, workers increasingly became exposed to the poison in arsenic mines, the number of which increased in the nineteenth century due to the rising demand for the mineral.

Organized arsenic production began in Britain when a tin smelting firm in Cornwall was used for the manufacture of arsenic trioxide in the early nineteenth century. By mid-century, as demand for arsenic grew, new plants were opened, some of which produced arsenic from arsenopyrite, a mineral that was abundantly available in Cornwall. As Andrew Meharg has noted, "From the arsenic factories fumes poured out night and day."[7]

By 1870, about half of the world's supply of arsenic was being produced by one mine in England, the Devon Great Consols. Devon was originally a copper mine, but when copper prices fell drastically in the 1860s, attention turned to a seemingly unimportant by-product, arsenic. One of the investors in the mine was William Morris, the famous artist and designer.[8]

By this time, the extraction of the ore involved mechanical drilling and blasting, which released large quantities of arsenic dust. However, the lives of these miners were already significantly affected by more general health problems such as silicosis (respiratory disease caused by dust), so it is not clear how much the exposure to arsenic was causing further damage to their health. Others working in the industry, however, were also affected. Grinders and millers of the ore would probably have inhaled or ingested some dust containing arsenic. Furnace operators were exposed to arsenic fumes.

The workers most affected by arsenic were those who shoveled the subli-mated arsenic oxide and those who packaged the product. The financial bur-dens incurred by the government under the Poor Laws due to these injuries raised concerns about the safety of these workers, and an investigation and subsequent report concluded that inadequate respiratory protection was resulting in excessive morbidity and mortality from lung disease among these men. A further study by the British Inspector of Factories and Inspector of Mines, however, minimized the hazards of the arsenic and blamed it on "the unhygienic practices of the workforce, especially with regard to cleanliness and the consumption of food." Declining demand for arsenic in the twentieth century eventually led to the end of the arsenic extraction industry in Britain.[9]

There remains a demand for arsenic in some industries, however, such as microelectronics, and arsenic is still encountered in the mining and extraction of other minerals. Therefore, cases of occupational arsenic poisoning have con-tinued to occur in recent times. A 1977 study of retired workers from a Japanese arsenic mine, for example, found symptoms of chronic arsenic poisoning, such as dermatitis and peripheral nervous disturbances, among the workers. Evidence also began to show that arsenic could cause lung cancer. Gold miners in Rhodesia, where there was arsenic in the gold ore, were found in 1957 to have higher than expected rates of lung cancer. In 1969 American investigators at the National Cancer Institute, studying workers at the Anaconda Smelter in Montana, provided convincing evidence that occupational exposure to arsenic was a factor in causing lung cancer. A 2008 paper examining lung cancer in copper smelter workers exposed to arsenic found that "inhalation of higher concentrations of arsenic over shorter durations was more deleterious than inhalation of lower concentrations over longer durations."[10]

Arsenic in the Artificial Flower Trade

Among arsenic's most important uses in the nineteenth century was its role as a coloring agent. The green color in paint, wallpaper, artificial flowers, and numerous other products was commonly produced with the aid of compounds such as copper arsenite (Scheele's green) and copper (II) acetoarsenite (Paris green). Those who worked in industries that used arsenic pigments often became victims of arsenic poisoning.

Among the products containing arsenic pigments were the artificial flowers, leaves, and fruits that became popular adornments for women's hats and clothing in Britain in the late 1850s.[11] More than ten thousand workers, most of them young women and girls, were employed in Britain as "artificial florists." Physician Arthur Hill Hassall, who had previously led a campaign against adulterated food and drinks, wrote about the health problems of the artificial florists in 1860 in *The Lancet*, a medical journal. He pointed out that the copper arsenite green pigment was inhaled by the workers and also irritated their skin. He described the symptoms of arsenic poisoning in two case histories and called for measures to protect the workers.

A popular article in the *Englishwoman's Journal* soon thereafter echoed Hassall's concerns and claimed that manufacturers lied to the workers by telling them that they did not employ arsenic pigments. The journal called upon women to discontinue their purchases of the green artificial flowers in order to eliminate the trade in these products.

A wider audience learned of the workers' plights when nineteen-year-old Matilda Scheurer, an artificial florist, died of arsenic poisoning in November 1861. An autopsy revealed that arsenic was present throughout her body, and the jury at the inquest returned a verdict of accidental death from copper arsenite. Her death was investigated by a health officer, who found that the factory where she had been employed was overcrowded and poorly ventilated. The women had not been informed that they were working with toxic materials. Some of the employees testified that they were constantly ill, a claim that was confirmed by a physician who had seen many of the women.

The health officer's report led to a broader government investigation into the use of copper arsenite in manufacturing processes, undertaken by William Guy, professor of forensic medicine at King's College, London. Although Guy became convinced that arsenic posed a threat to the health of the artificial florists, he did not feel justified in recommending the prohibition of copper arsenite in manufacturing. As historian P. W. J. Bartrip wrote, "Such an approach was, of course, consistent with the principle of *laissez-faire* whereby adult employees were perceived to be equal participants in the market place with their employers. If they preferred not to pursue a hazardous occupation they were free to shun it and take alternative employment."[12]

In reality, of course, many of the workers were not in a position to quit their jobs and find employment elsewhere. As one person commented about an industry in which arsenic was employed, "The workers generally dread the occupation, but dread still more the alternative of being without work."[13]

Some employers did begin to voluntarily provide the workers with gauze masks, but they were uncomfortably warm, and many women refused to wear them. Some of the women did try to employ makeshift masks using their aprons or a layer of muslin, but a loosely tied sheet of fabric was not an effective shield against the poisonous particles in the air.

By 1865, however, the use of copper arsenite in the artificial flower trade appears to have become much less common in Britain. An investigator for the Children's Employment Commission reported that he had found that arsenical colors were rarely used any longer in the trade. Even a London physician who was somewhat skeptical of these claims had to admit that arsenic use in the trade had declined and that he had not seen a case of arsenic poisoning in quite some time. Changes in fashion, with more sober colors than the bright green produced by arsenic pigments coming into favor, may also have played a role in the decreased use of arsenic in the trade.

Paint and Wallpaper

Arsenic pigments were also used to color paint and wallpaper. By the 1850s several physicians and chemists had warned of the possible dangers of wallpaper

containing arsenic, generally used to produce a vivid green color. Soon after
it was established in 1862, the Children's Employment Commission decided
that paper staining was one of the trades that required prompt attention.[14]
The assistant commissioner charged with conducting the investigation was
physician Henry Lord, the same man who had investigated the artificial
flower trade for the commission. Lord studied 26 firms with an estimated
1,750 to 1,850 employees, the majority of whom (1,150) were children or young
persons. More than half of this latter group were under the age of thirteen,
with the youngest being eight. Over 80 percent of the children and young
persons were male.

Lord found that the factories were hot and had an unwholesome atmosphere. The work involved long hours, resulting in fatigue and poor health.
Bartrip described the work as follows: "The trade consisted of printing
coloured patterns or designs on paper. This was done either by hand, using
blocks, or mechanically, by means of steam-driven rollers. The colouring matter comprised emerald green [Paris green] 'in greater or less proportions.'"[15]

Oddly enough, Lord did not mention the dangers of emerald green in his
report. The commission reviewed his evidence and concluded that the
arsenic pigment was dangerous only if "it had been poorly manufactured and
was, in consequence, powdery; if it had been imperfectly mixed with size
(adhesive); if the workers were exposed for too long; or if cleanliness was not
observed."[16] They also believed that precautions were being taken in the factories to protect the workers and noted that reported serious cases of poisoning were rare. They thus decided that there was no need for special
legislation or regulations to protect workers from emerald green. Although
the Factory Acts that provided some regulation of industry did not apply to
the paper staining trade, the commission optimistically anticipated that the
acts would be extended to encompass the trade, providing some oversight
over conditions that might lead to poisoning.

Bartrip has pointed out that the commission based their findings solely
on the documentation provided by Lord, who had paid almost no attention
to the emerald green problem in his report. They relied largely on transcripts
of interviews that Lord had conducted with workers, managers, and owners.
Bartrip rightly concluded that the employees, whose interviews were not
anonymous, were hardly likely to have been completely honest in their

comments on the health standards in the factories. Of course, managers and owners were also unlikely to have been critical of conditions in the workplace. In addition, with one exception, Lord had failed to interview technical experts such as chemists and physicians. In spite of these flaws in methodology, Lord's information did provide some evidence of arsenic toxicity that the commission essentially ignored. Bartrip stated that "comparison of the report with the full transcript of evidence suggests that, deliberately or fortuitously, the commissioners underplayed the arsenic problem, justifying this by means of selective quotation and omission."[17]

Workers who manufactured the pigments were also at risk. A report in the *British Medical Journal* in 1893 discussed the dangers of the arsenical dust created in the production of emerald green, which covered the workers and was no doubt inhaled by them. The article noted that it was obvious that skin problems caused by arsenic were prevalent among the workers, and concluded that the work was more generally injurious to their health. It added, "It is curious that so little medical evidence should be available regarding the frequency of arsenical poisoning among the workers at these colours, but it must be remembered that the more men recognise their trade as the cause of their troubles the less likely are they to go to the doctor while they know the cause persists. They hardly in fact look on their condition as a disease, but regard it as an unavoidable hardship attaching to their occupation."[18]

The *Journal* went on to explain, however, that the Home Secretary had just issued regulations for processes involved in the manufacture of paints and colors and in the extraction of arsenic. These regulations mandated that employers must provide workers with facilities and supplies for washing their hands and face, respirators and suitable clothing, and any necessary medicines. They also had to ensure that no food was eaten in any part of the works. Employees were also instructed to wear the respirators and special clothing, to wash before meals and before leaving the facility, and not to eat or smoke in the works.

Workers who used arsenic pigments to color paint, as well as those who applied paint, also might have suffered from arsenic poisoning. An interesting case is that of artists, who often made use of arsenic pigments. Ramazzini had already included a chapter on the diseases of painters in his classic book on occupational health. Given the various oils and chemicals that they applied in their art, Ramazzini was not surprised that the painters he knew were almost all sickly and that history showed that famous painters tended not to have long lives. Although he did not specifically mention arsenic, he did refer to the poisonous nature of the various minerals that they used. The artists favored these minerals because "the Metallick Colours are much more durable than those of a vegetable Extraction."[19] In his important book on occupational diseases in the 1830s, Thackrah did specifically mention the poisonous effects of "mineral green" (Scheele's green) on painters (including house painters) and paper stainers.[20] Several years before the appearance of Thackrah's book, an anonymous publication entitled *The Painter's and Varnisher's Pocket Manual* discussed the various poisons to which painters and varnishers are exposed, including arsenic.[21]

Arsenic pigments have been used since ancient times in painting and decorative arts. For example, orpiment and realgar have been found on ancient Egyptian papyri and Greek artifacts. Orpiment gives a yellow color and realgar an orange-red color. In fact, arsenic pigments have been used in painting in a broad array of cultures, from medieval Persia to seventeenth- and eighteenth-century South America. These pigments were widely used by European and American artists as well. A study of the illnesses of several great masters, including Rubens and Renoir, argued that exposure to heavy metals (including arsenic) in their paints contributed to their health problems. The article pointed out that some artists licked their brushes (presumably to point them) and probably often did not wash their hands before eating or hand rolling cigarettes, thus ingesting toxins. There is no clear way of knowing, however, how many artists may have suffered ill effects from the use of orpiment and realgar pigments, as well as from the later use of Scheele's green and Paris green.[22]

Taxidermy

Another occupation that exposed its workers to arsenic was the field of taxidermy, the art of preserving and mounting dead animals for display. Animal skins have been tanned for clothing and shelter since ancient times. During the Age of Exploration following the discovery of the New World, travelers and explorers began to bring back live animals from exotic locales to Europe. When these animals died, collectors and naturalists sought methods to preserve their bodies for study and exhibition in both the increasing number of natural history museums and the so-called cabinets of curiosity assembled by collectors. At first, the bodies were simply skinned, wired and mounted, or sometimes stuffed with cotton or straw. Various spices were used in some cases as preservatives (and perhaps to mask unpleasant odors as well). But relatively few specimens lasted for more than about thirty years before they decomposed or were consumed by insects.[23]

The French naturalist René-Antoine Ferchault de Réamur complained in the eighteenth century about the inadequacy of the methods available for preserving animals, especially birds. Such methods as stuffing the bird's body with fabric or hay, or using aromatic spices or a drying agent such as alum to embalm the specimen, did not protect against insects. Naturalists searched for a better preservative that would successfully resist insect attacks. Toxic substances such as mercury and arsenic were also tried.

Arsenic had been used to some extent in tanning and as a pesticide, but it was the arsenical soap developed by the French apothecary and naturalist Jean-Baptiste Bécoeur that made it a staple of taxidermy. Bécoeur apparently developed this preparation around the middle of the nineteenth century. Since he was intent on making money from his invention, he refused to reveal its composition during his lifetime. In order to advertise his product, he attempted to have specimens preserved with it placed on display in various collections. After his death, it was revealed that his product was a mixture of powdered white arsenic, soap, salt of tartar (potassium carbonate), camphor, and powdered lime (a mineral composed of different calcium salts). Bécoeur's arsenical soap was eventually widely adopted by taxidermists and largely solved their preservation problems. Commenting on the taxidermy literature of the nineteenth and early twentieth centuries, Paul Farber wrote: "A review of that literature shows that instead of laments over the sad state of ornithological [bird] collections, as appeared in the eighteenth century, one finds dozens of treatises confidently describing methods of preserving birds—practically all of which recommend Bécoeur's soap or some variation on it. The collectors of the nineteenth century, then, no longer regarded taxidermy as a problem but considered it a technique."[24]

An article in the *American Naturalist* in 1869 described in detail the use of both powdered arsenic and arsenical soap in the preservation of animal skins, and it also provided instructions for the preparation of the soap. The author emphasized that salt, alum, and spices should only be used when arsenic could not be obtained, for these substances were by no means substitutes for arsenic.[25]

The field of taxidermy blossomed in the nineteenth century thanks to the passion of the Victorians for collecting and cataloging. As Stephen Asma noted, "If one wanted to be a Victorian naturalist of any distinction, one had to be well versed in the taxidermic arts." Darwin, for example, learned taxidermy from a freed black slave who worked at the Edinburgh Museum of Science and Art, one of many institutions that employed taxidermists by this time. In the United States as well, interest in natural history burgeoned in the nineteenth century, leading to an expansion of the field of taxidermy. Most large American urban areas had at least one taxidermy shop.[26]

Arsenic was used for preserving specimens in museum collections around the world at least until the 1980s, and in some cases beyond. Dr. Walter Hough, head curator of the Anthropology Department of the Smithsonian Institutions' National Museum of Natural History, made extensive use of various arsenic preparations for pest eradication and management in the collections in his charge from the 1880s possibly through his retirement in 1935. He recommended that specimens treated with arsenic or other toxic substances carry labels printed with a skull and the word "poisoned." In many cases, however, arsenic-treated museum specimens in various collections are not identified as being potentially toxic. Because of the large number of museum specimens (especially in natural history collections) that were prepared with arsenic, curators and others who handle the specimens have been warned to take appropriate preventive measures against arsenic poisoning.[27] Writing in 2008, William R. Cullen reported: "Many objects on display in the City of Vancouver Museum were recently found to have high amounts of arsenic compounds on their surface and some of these came from the part of the collection that was open to the public, especially to children, for hands-on examination. The exhibit was rapidly rearranged."[28]

It is difficult to say how many people in the taxidermy or museum professions suffered from arsenic poisoning over the decades. Many cases no

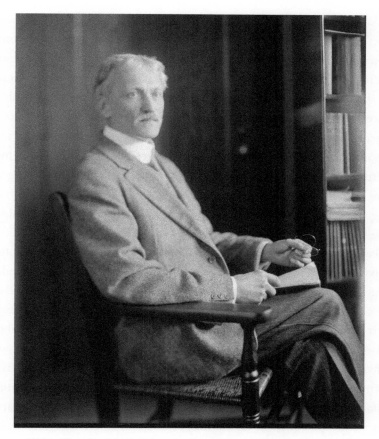

**Walter Hough of the Smithsonian Institution made extensive use of
arsenic preparations for pest eradication and management of the specimens
in the collections under his charge.** *Courtesy of the Library of Congress.*

doubt were unrecognized or unreported. Arsenic has been shown to be carcinogenic, but cancer would likely not show up for many years and would not necessarily be associated with arsenic exposure. Some naturalists and taxidermists did express concerns about the possible hazards of using arsenic in their work. The French chemist J. N. Gannal, when discussing the preservation of specimens by taxidermy, wrote in his 1836 book on embalming: "Some naturalists, fearful of the daily use of arsenic, have endeavoured to replace their preservative by another composition, but have never succeeded in obtaining results equally advantageous."[29]

Although taxidermy was often listed as one of the occupations whose practitioners were exposed to arsenic, there is little quantitative data on the subject. One paper published as recently as 1995 by researchers in Denmark, where arsenic was still being used in the preservation of animal specimens, did show that urine arsenic levels in the taxidermists in the study was almost twice as high as the reference level. However, it is not clear what effects this concentration had on the workers, and the sample size (thirteen) was small. Among the cases of arsenic poisoning reported to the Chief Inspector of Factories in London for the period 1900–1913 were three individuals who were described as "sorting bird skins" and one who was involved with tanning. Most taxidermists did not work in factories, however, and so would not have been included in such reports.[30]

Pat Morris of the Department of Zoology at the Royal Holloway College, University of London, published a study in 1982 in which he examined the longevity of a group of taxidermists using historical data. Morris noted that since taxidermists worked with arsenic and other poisons, one might expect their longevity to be lower than normal. Although little biographical data is available on most taxidermists, Morris was able to identify thirty-two individuals from the late nineteenth and early twentieth centuries for whom birth and death dates were available in S. Herriott's *British Taxidermists: A Historical Directory* and C. Frost's *Victorian Taxidermy*. He found that the average lifespan of these taxidermists was about seventy-six years, which was better than average for the period. Morris concluded, perhaps half in jest, "Perhaps their occupational hazards were not so dire after all? In fact contrary to expectation, this analysis might even suggest that poisons were good for you; maybe arsenic preserves lives as well as skins! Or maybe the old taxidermists were just happy in their work. Contentment is surely one of the best antidotes to old age, and discontent a greater threat to Health and Safety than mere chemicals."[31]

Morris's study, however, is hardly conclusive. His sample size was relatively small and not randomly selected. His investigation was also limited to the question of longevity, and did not examine the overall health of the taxidermists. Nonetheless, some taxidermists were not convinced that arsenic was all that harmful to them. Noted taxidermist Bruce Schwendeman, for example, was quoted recently in a book by Melissa Milgrom as saying that "Arsenic is an overrated poison!" In fact, Bruce Schwendeman and his father, David, in speaking with Milgrom, attributed the longevity of David's mother, who was ninety-four at the time of her death, to arsenic exposure. They claimed that "she stored it in her fatty tissues and reabsorbed it as she aged."[32]

Probably the most famous possible victim of arsenic poisoning from taxidermy work is the artist Raphaelle Peale, who assumed the post of taxidermist at his father's natural history museum in 1798. Art historian Phoebe Lloyd, collaborating with physician Gordon Bendersky, challenged the common view that Peale's chronic illness and ultimate death at the age of fifty-one were the result of heavy drinking, suggesting instead that the cause of his health problems was exposure to arsenic (and probably also mercury) over many years of preparing specimens for his father's museum. Their conclusions were based largely on a document from Raphaelle's nephew, who speculated on the toxic effect of the taxidermy chemicals on his uncle, and on the symptoms of the latter's illness. Raphaelle himself believed that arsenic was to blame for his suffering. Lloyd and Bendersky also argued that Charles Willson Peale was aware of the hazards that his son faced in his taxidermy work but ignored them. In fact, they claimed that the father did not even make available to his son an antidote to arsenic that he had recorded in his own diary. They commented: "Over the next twenty-three years, Charles Willson proved persuasive in driving his firstborn to an extremely hazardous task, imputed the subsequent symptoms to gout and excessive drink, avoided mention of arsenic and mercury in his correspondence, and impugned his son's reputation."[33]

Even before this paper was published, however, it stimulated controversy. Lillian Miller, editor of the Peale family papers, read galley proofs of the Lloyd-Bendersky paper and challenged their conclusions. In an interview reported in the *New York Times*, she argued that it was wrong to ascribe malicious motives to Charles Willson Peale: "She added that several members of the Peale family worked with the taxidermic chemicals without suffering ill effects; that Raphaelle did not work at the museum as long as the others; that there is no proof that the elder Peale kept the antidote from Raphaelle, and that Raphaelle was a known alcoholic who frequently had to be carried home from taverns."[34]

The debate culminated in a special feature in the *Transactions and Studies of the College of Physicians of Philadelphia* in 1994, where both sides had their

say. Lloyd and Miller, in adjacent articles, responded to each other's criti-
cisms and provided additional evidence to support their points of view. For
example, Miller pointed out that another physician, Gerald Weissmann, had
published an editorial that contradicted the diagnosis of arsenic and mercury
poisoning for Raphaelle, concluding that the symptoms seemed more like
those of lead poisoning, which he believed resulted from drinking alcoholic
beverages distilled or stored in lead-lined containers. Lloyd defended her
position, but admitted that the question of Raphaelle's death, which was
officially attributed to consumption, had not been put to rest. She suggested
that the only solution was to exhume the corpse and look for evidence of
arsenic and mercury poisoning. This step, however, has not been taken, so
the cause of Peale's death remains controversial.[35]

Embalming

Efforts to preserve human corpses go back to the mummification procedures
of ancient Egypt. Other cultures, such as the Incas of Peru, also practiced
mummification. The preparation of mummies was generally done for reli-
gious purposes, to preserve the body for the afterlife. Although chemicals
such as natron (a mixture of sodium salts) in Egypt were used to dessicate
(dry out) the body, climate conditions also helped preserve the corpse in
some countries. For example, the extremely dry climate of Egypt and the
low temperatures and humidity of the underground tombs of Han dynasty–
era China played a major role in the preservation of corpses.

Embalming techniques appear to have been first used in Europe in the late
Middle Ages. Generally the bodies embalmed for funeral purposes were those
of royalty or other dignitaries. During the Crusades, interest in embalming
increased as crusading noblemen often wished to have their bodies transported from the Holy Land for burial at home in Europe. The embalming
techniques of the period were fairly crude, generally involving removal of the
internal organs and stuffing the body with herbs to reduce putrefaction. In
the sixteenth century, improvements were made in embalming techniques
with the introduction in Europe of balms, ointments, and powders to dehy-
drate and dry out the corpse. At about this same time, the practice of anatomical embalming, intended to preserve the body for anatomists and naturalists

for research and teaching purposes (as opposed to preserving bodies for view-
ing at a funeral), was also introduced. Most embalming at the time was done
by physicians and surgeons.

Modern embalming techniques involve the injection of preservative
chemicals into the blood vessels. The method was first explored by anatomists by the sixteenth century. For example, Leonardo da Vinci and William
Harvey experimented with arterial injections in an effort to preserve corpses
for anatomical investigation. Lodewijk de Bils introduced a technique of
preservation involving the injection of a wax-like substance into the blood
vessels in the 1650s. Fellow Dutchman Frederik Ruysch popularized the procedure and is sometimes credited with being the first person to embalm by
injecting a preservative chemical solution into the blood vessels. The composition of his solution is unknown.[36]

Arsenic appears to have been first introduced into embalming fluids
around the turn of the nineteenth century. It was already well known that
arsenic could preserve animal matter, as has been noted in the above discussion about taxidermy. Physicians had also commented upon the fact that the
bodies of persons who had died of arsenic poisoning decomposed more
slowly than normal. In the early nineteenth century, physicians and chemists
were experimenting with new processes and chemical solutions for preserving
bodies for scientific research. Three men—a chemist and two physicians—
were particularly instrumental in the development of chemical embalming.

> In France, the chemist J. N. Gannal (1791–1852) earned his place among
> the famous figures connected with embalming innovation in the 19th
> century, alongside two of his contemporaries—Italian physician G.
> Tranchina and French physician J. P. Sucquet. Considered as the fathers
> of modern embalming methods, their processes exploited the potential
> alliance between the chemist and the physician, combining chemical
> solutions and arterial injection. Their research was not restricted to sci-
> entific and medical activities but also covered funeral embalming, using
> simplified methods that did not lacerate the corpse.[37]

Gannal's formula for his embalming fluid included arsenic as one of the
ingredients. Tranchina also used arsenic in his process. While the arsenic was

effective for preservation purposes, concerns were soon raised that embalming with arsenic might interfere with criminal prosecutions. The legal community in France petitioned for a ban on the use of arsenic in embalming because it could interfere with murder investigations involving arsenical poisoning. Defense attorneys could argue that any arsenic found in an analysis of an embalmed corpse was the result of embalming, rather than poisoning. France did prohibit the use of arsenic in embalming in 1846, but it continued to be used in other countries.

Arsenic embalming became common in the United States during the Civil War. The demand for the preservation of corpses grew during the war, as many families wanted the remains of their loved ones transported home for funerals and burial. The practice of exhibiting the embalmed corpse became popular in the United States during and after the war, introducing a new model for funerals. The key figure in Civil War embalming was Dr. Thomas Holmes (1817–1900).

Holmes was born in New York City, and, although he studied medicine, it is not clear if he ever graduated. He practiced medicine and serve as a coroner's physician in New York City and later in Brooklyn in the 1850s. During this time, he experimented with different chemicals for embalming, including Gannal's solution. He was asked by the War Department to assist with the embalming of dead soldiers. He trained American surgeons accompanying the troops onto the battlefield to perform embalming and helped set up partnerships between embalming surgeons and undertakers. Holmes also sold his embalming fluid, whose composition he kept secret. Arsenic, however, was a key ingredient.

Holmes also set up an embalming practice in Washington, D.C., during the war. He claims to have ultimately prepared about four thousand bodies, although this number could be an exaggeration. Among his "clients" were eight generals. When the Civil War ended, he returned to Brooklyn, where he only occasionally did any embalming, though he continued to sell his embalming fluid. Other civilian embalmers also set up business to embalm soldiers during the war.[38]

As suggested above, the practice of embalming of bodies for funeral display became increasingly common in the period after the Civil War, especially in the United States. The function of embalming was also passed from physicians to undertakers. As Trompette and Lemonnier explained:

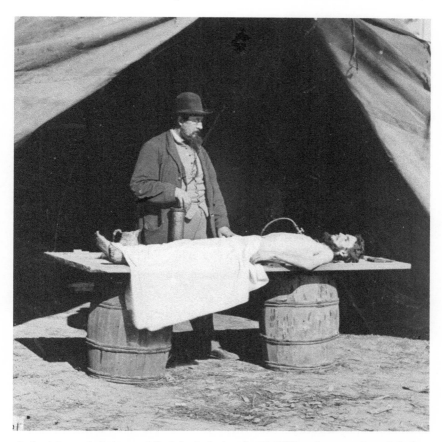

A physician embalming a soldier's body during the Civil War, when arsenic embalming fluids became popular in the United States. *Courtesy of the Library of Congress.*

Funeral historians agree that the American Civil War marked a turning point in "The American Way of Death," notably in terms of the legitimization and democratization of embalming for body display. Underlying this Cultural Revolution, the activity of the embalming physicians fostered the commercial development of embalming (techniques, fluids, instruments, etc.), which was soon to be taken over by undertakers with whom they had set up alliances. Over the following decades, the professional embalming map was redrawn as physicians were more or less removed and an increasing number of embalming chemical companies appeared.[39]

Arsenic became the primary ingredient in the early commercial embalming fluids and remained so until the early twentieth century. Cullen has noted that "the amount used per body was in the range of 110 grams to 6 kilograms, and it very effectively killed the micro-organisms responsible for decomposition. The treated bodies were relatively supple and could be easily dressed and positioned."[40]

Embalmed bodies, such as those of notorious criminals, and mummies (both real and fake) were also sometimes exhibited at side shows, carnivals, and dime museums. One of the most famous of these was Elmer McCurdy, a bank and train robber who was shot to death by lawmen in Oklahoma in 1911. His body was taken to a funeral home, where it was embalmed with an arsenic solution. No one claimed the body, and the undertaker refused to give it up until he had been paid for his work. The corpse was well preserved, and the undertaker decided to exhibit it to make money. He dressed the corpse, placed a rifle in its hand, and then proceeded to allow people to view the body for a nickel. A man claiming to be Elmer's brother took the body in 1916, ostensibly to bury it. However, Elmer soon turned up in a carnival show as an exhibit called "The Outlaw Who Would Never Be Captured." Elmer continued to be exhibited on and off over the following decades and even made a brief appearance in the film *She Freak* (1967). He showed up again at an amusement park in California in the 1970s. By this time, Elmer was thought to be a dummy until an arm broke off when he was being moved in 1976, revealing bone and ending the corpse's career.[41]

Some medical professionals expressed concerns about the possible ill effects of arsenical embalming fluids on the health of physicians, morticians, and others who practiced the art. For example, Gannal commented on the potential hazards of Tranchini's embalming fluid, which consisted of two pounds of arsenic in twenty pounds of water or alcohol, in his 1836 treatise: "I think that the employment of this method presents real dangers for the anatomist, of which the following is a proof: Doctor Poirson declared before the Academy of Medicine, that he had been exceedingly incommoded, as well as two of his colleagues, in having embalmed two generals with this substance; he attributed this derangement of his health to the arsenic absorbed during the preparation."[42]

Gannal went on to mention that the corpse and the table on which it lay were covered with dead flies. He speculated that the flies might have been killed by "arsenical hydrogen" (arsine, or arsenic trihydride) gas given off by the corpse. As noted previously, arsenic was also one of the ingredients in Gannal's embalming solution but in much smaller amounts. It appears that Gannal did not initially reveal that his formula contained arsenic, and supposedly, when physicians learned of this fact, they were outraged and pressed for the passage of the 1846 law banning the use of arsenic in embalming fluids. There is even a story, which has apparently never been conclusively documented as fact, that Gannal had to reveal the presence of arsenic in his embalming fluid on the stand in court in order to save the life of a woman accused of murdering her husband when arsenic was found in the body of the deceased (who had been embalmed by Gannal).[43]

Another example of a warning about the dangers of arsenic was issued in Carl Lewis Barnes's 1898 book on *The Art and Science of Embalming*. He noted that the embalmer handles fluids containing large amounts of poison such as arsenic and mercury and that he "will soon learn whether his system is capable of resisting the absorption of such chemicals." If he is susceptible to the action of arsenic, then by constant exposure to a fluid containing the chemical, he will suffer from chronic arsenic poisoning.[44]

The toxic effect of arsenic on embalmers has also been cited by various authors as one of the reasons why its use for preserving bodies was eventually abandoned.[45] However, it would appear that concern over the interference of this practice with murder investigations involving arsenic poisoning was at least as important a reason for the abandonment of arsenic embalming fluids. Articles in the medical literature opposing the practice generally stressed the problems that arsenic embalming created for forensic science. Some writers pointed that, in addition to allowing murderers to go free, embalming could possibly lead to the conviction for arsenic poisoning of innocent persons in cases where an arsenic embalming fluid had been used on the deceased without the knowledge of the court.[46]

One medical examiner wrote to the *Boston Medical and Surgical Journal* in 1890 protesting the practice of embalming, which he called "one of the greatest evils with which the medical examiner has to deal in the discharge of his duties." He called for legislation that would require a physician's certificate of the cause of death, approved by the Board of Health, before anybody could be embalmed. He described a case in which he was convinced that the deceased had been poisoned with arsenic but which was dropped by prosecutors when they learned that an arsenical fluid had been used to embalm the body before the autopsy was conducted, and he complained that "this is, I believe, only one of many cases where the ends of justice are defeated, and all chances of detecting poisons (i.e., the most common arsenic and corrosive sublimate) rendered impossible by the process of embalming."[47]

As in the case of taxidermists, there does not appear to be any quantitative data documenting the extent of the effects of arsenic on the health or longevity of embalmers. By the early twentieth century, however, arsenic was being eliminated from embalming fluids in the United States. Michigan appears to have been the first state to ban its use in embalming around the turn of the twentieth century. Other states soon followed suit, and by 1920 arsenic was no longer being used in embalming.[48] Rather, it was replaced by formaldehyde, the preserving ability of which was discovered in the 1890s. By the beginning of the twentieth century, formalin (a stable solution of formaldehyde in methanol) became available at a cheap enough price to make it economical to use it in place of arsenic. By the 1990s, some companies were replacing formaldehyde with other chemicals in their embalming fluids because health and environmental concerns had been raised by then about the dangers of formaldehyde, as various studies had suggested that it was carcinogenic.[49] Formaldehyde embalming fluid also was used, generally in combination with other drugs such as marijuana, as a mind-altering drug beginning in the 1980s.[50]

Although embalmers were the workers most directly affected by arsenic embalming fluids, there were other individuals who also came into contact with these fluids. For example, bodies provided to medical schools for dissection, or to medical examiners for autopsy, sometimes had been embalmed with arsenic. To cite one instance, medical student John Snow, who would later become famous for his investigation of cholera, wrote to a British medical journal in the 1830s warning of the potential dangers of cadavers. He reported that he and fellow students had dissected several bodies treated with arsenic and had suffered from vomiting on each occasion. But historian James Whorton, author of The Arsenic Century, has stated that he found no reports of human fatalities caused by working on arsenic-preserved corpses.[51]

The presence of arsenic in bodies can sometimes present problems today to archaeologists and cemetery workers who handle human remains. As John Konefes and Michael McGee warned in 1996, arsenic poisoning could result from hand contact with dust or objects containing arsenic, with subsequent hand-to-mouth contact. Arsenic dust could also settle on objects that later come into contact with the mouth, such as soda cans and cigarettes. Arsenic dust could also be inhaled, and contact with the skin could result in severe irritation. They concluded, "Due to the level of toxicity associated with arsenic, it is important to take precautionary measures when working in and around burial sites that may contain arsenic embalmed remains. Protective measures include protective work clothing and equipment, housekeeping, and hygiene practices."[52]

Other Occupations

Given the ubiquitous presence of arsenic in so many products in the nineteenth (and even into the twentieth) century, it is not surprising that it presented hazards in other industries as well. In any situation where one had to work in frequent contact with arsenic, the potential for poisoning was present.

One example of an occupation where arsenic poisoning was not uncommon was sheep dressing, especially in Britain, where the production of wool was an important industry. In order to protect the health of their sheep, farmers would periodically treat the animals with preparations designed to kill lice, ticks, and other parasites. Although not all of these "dips" contained arsenic, the great majority of them did. Workers involved in the manufacture of sheep dip were covered under British factory law, but those who worked on the farms were not. The dressing routine involved immersing a sheep in a vat of the dip for about a minute. Workers unavoidably came into contact with the arsenic mixture. Whorton has described the process:

The procedure was not one in which the animals were inclined to cooperate, of course, so the dipper was forced to wrap his arms around the sheep and hold it close against his body while working the liquid into the wool with his hands. His clothing was soon saturated with the mixture, its penetration to the skin guaranteed by "the friction which must be caused by a living sheep half drowned in poison, trying to struggle out for its life." An efficient dipper would dress more than a hundred sheep a day.[53]

The areas on the workers' bodies most affected were the hands, forearms, and scrotum. The smart workers wore a leather apron and washed the genitals at the end of the day, as failure to do so generally resulted in painful blistering of the testicles. In general, skin irritation was common among these workers, and the dip could also be absorbed into their bodies, resulting in constitutional poisoning.[54]

Farm workers who handled pesticides were also often at risk for arsenic poisoning in the late nineteenth and first half of the twentieth century, as compounds such as Paris green, London purple (monocalcium arsenite) and lead arsenate were widely used as pesticides in this period, especially in the United States. As late as 1945, half of the arsenious oxide produced in the United States went into the preparation of agricultural pesticides.[55]

Workers using the pesticides on farms were particularly at risk for getting the chemical on their skin, leading to contact dermatitis and potentially skin cancer (which might not show up for decades). There have been numerous reports in the literature of cancer, liver damage, and other health problems among vineyard workers as well. Gardeners also were exposed to arsenical compounds, and there were reports in the literature of accidental poisonings of garden staff by London purple. Kipling stated that between 1946 and 1955, there were an estimated fifty deaths a year in agriculture in the United States from arsenic poisoning. Inorganic arsenic pesticides were essentially abandoned in the 1950s in favor of the newly discovered dichlorodiphenyltrichloroethane (DDT), but organic arsenic compounds are still selectively used as herbicides.[56]

Because of its pesticide properties, arsenic has also been used for over a hundred years as a preservative in the treatment of wood. Workers involved in impregnating the wood, and some of those who later handle it (e.g., sawmill workers), are exposed to various arsenic compounds. Several studies have demonstrated an increased risk of cancer in woodworkers who handle arsenic-impregnated products. Some have also expressed concerns about the exposure of consumers (especially children) to arsenic-treated wood, most commonly containing chromated copper arsenate (CCA), on playgrounds, decks, and other sites, and the manufacture of such wood for residential use ended as of December 31, 2003, through an agreement between manufacturers and the Environmental Protection Agency.[57]

Certain industrial processes can also lead to the release of arsine (arsenic trihydride), a colorless, flammable, and highly toxic gas. It has a garlicky odor, but the smell is an unreliable indicator of danger, as toxic effects can occur below the odor threshold. One textbook of environmental health and toxicology has stated that "arsine gas exposure usually occurs in the industrial-occupational setting, which includes smelting and refining of metals and ores, galvanizing, soldering, etching, lead plating, metallurgy, burning of fossil fuels, and microelectronic semiconductor production." The primary toxic effect of arsine is due to its ability to bind with red blood cells and cause them to lyse (disintegrate).[58]

Workers in various other industries have also been exposed to arsenic. For example, arsenic has been used in such industries as glassmaking, tanning, and the manufacture of lead shot, rat poison, and many other products. The widespread use of arsenic historically resulted in exposure to this poisonous substance not only among workers but among the public as they came into contact with resulting products.

CHAPTER FOUR

The Ubiquitous Element
Arsenic in the Environment

Although the uses for arsenic were limited before about 1800, the employment of arsenic compounds exploded in the nineteenth century, which medical historian James Whorton has dubbed the "arsenic century." Arsenic found a host of uses in the home, on the farm, and in various industries during this time period. Whorton summarized the situation with respect to the ubiquitous presence of arsenic as follows:

> A great deal of it was introduced purposely into many of the components of everyday life, with the result that people took it in with fruits and vegetables, swallowed it with wine, inhaled it from cigarettes, absorbed it from cosmetics, and imbibed it even from the pint glass. . . . The substance was present in a broad assortment of household items from candies and candles to cookware, concert tickets, and preserved partridge heads used to ornament ladies headdresses. . . . Christmas tree ornaments and children's stuffed animals, no less, were often arsenical, and the money used to purchase all these products was itself sometimes contaminated.[1]

Another medical historian, Peter Bartrip, also listed some of the many Victorian goods that contained arsenic: "These included clothes, soap, books, kitchen-ware, glass and glassware, paint and distemper, artificial and dried flowers, stuffed animals, playing cards, paper and packaging, candles, handkerchiefs, fly-papers, lampshades, soft-furnishings, artificial leaves and fruit, patent medicine, and wallpaper."[2]

Not surprisingly, the presence of arsenic in so many products in the nineteenth century resulted in many people suffering from unintentional arsenic poisoning. It was not only the workers involved in industrial processes involving arsenic who were subject to the chemical's poisonous effects but the consumers who used arsenic-impregnated articles. As Whorton noted, "Whether at home amidst arsenical curtains and papers, or at play swirling about the papered, curtained ballroom in arsenical gowns and gloves, no one was beyond the poison's reach."[3]

Not all arsenic in the environment comes from man-made sources, however. Significant quantities of the metal occur naturally. Arsenic is widely distributed in the Earth's crust, existing in over 150 different minerals. It is estimated that about one-third of the arsenic in the atmosphere comes from natural sources, primarily volcanoes. Nevertheless, the great majority of arsenic in the environment is a result of human activity, such as metal mining and smelting, pesticide use, wood combustion, and waste incineration. Most of this arsenic is released into land or soil, but substantial amounts are also released to air and water.

Deadly Shades of Green

Workers involved in the manufacture of arsenical pigments and in the use of these substances for coloring wallpaper, artificial flowers, and other products often fell victim to arsenic poisoning. But what of these products once they left the factory and entered the home? Before the late eighteenth century, green color was usually produced by copper compounds that did not give a very intense hue. The introduction of arsenical pigments such as Scheele's green and Paris green in the late eighteenth and the first half of the nineteenth century, however, provided manufacturers of colored articles with much more intense and bright green colors. Methods were developed to produce various shades of green from these pigments, which quickly came to dominate the market for green colors. About seven hundred tons of Scheele's green was manufactured in England alone in 1860. Arsenical pigments were used to some extent in other colors as well.[4]

By the middle of the nineteenth century, shades of green had become especially fashionable, particularly for women's clothing and home furnishings. Green paints were applied to walls, as well as to items ranging from shelves to Venetian blinds to children's toys. Paint would often flake off or be accidentally rubbed off walls and other surfaces. Arsenical dust could then be inhaled or paint chips ingested by young children. Paint on toys was often loosely applied and easily removed, especially by children putting the toys in their mouths. The noted British toxicologist Alfred Taylor reported that he noticed patches of green on the lower crust of a loaf of bread that he had purchased. He analyzed the green material and found it to consist of Scheele's green. Upon inquiry, he discovered that the green paint had recently been used to cover the shelves on which the baker placed his bread.[5]

There were numerous reports of arsenic poisoning resulting from contact with common household items in the literature. In the early 1880s, for example, the Medical Society of London investigated the matter by sending a series of questionnaires to medical practitioners throughout England. They received over one hundred reports of arsenical poisoning in the domestic environment, including thirty-six cases involving wallpaper and five involving wall paint. There were also reports of poisoning due to clothing, artificial flowers, toys, and other products. Another study cited similar cases, as well as arsenic poisoning due to book covers, playing cards, and the lining of a baby's bassinet.[6]

Green arsenic–colored artificial flowers and women's clothing became extremely popular around the middle of the nineteenth century. Given that clothing was worn next to the skin, the potential for toxic effects was significant. Green muslin ball gowns were very much in fashion, colored with loosely applied arsenic dyes. A London physician wrote in the *Times* about the dangers posed by green muslin gowns, wondering "what the atmosphere of a ball room must be where these muslin fabrics are worn, and where the agitation of skirts consequent on dancing must be constantly discharging arsenical poison."[7]

Several European countries such as France, Sweden, and the German states of Prussia and Bavaria enacted legislation prohibiting the importation or sale of certain articles colored with arsenic pigments, such as wallpaper, in the nineteenth century. In England and the United States, however, strong traditions of free enterprise and laissez-faire government prevented the placement of any significant restrictions on the manufacture and sale of such products. One British medical journal, *The Lancet*, complained that the government respected freedom in trade to the point of allowing the poisoning of the nation's children by arsenical products.[8]

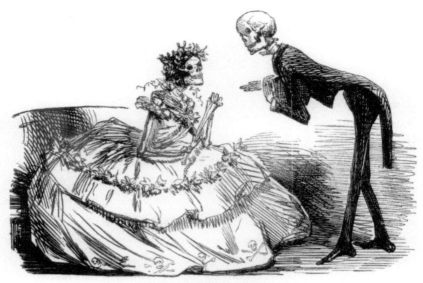

THE ARSENIC WALTZ.

THE NEW DANCE OF DEATH. (DEDICATED TO THE GREEN WREATH AND DRESS-MONGERS.)

"The Arsenic Waltz," a cartoon referring to the new "Dance of Death" resulting from the use of fabrics colored green by arsenic pigments. *From* Punch, *February 8, 1862.*

The product that probably caused the most concern on the part of the medical profession and the public was arsenical wallpaper, which increased dramatically in popularity in the Victorian era due to a number of factors. In Britain, for example, decreases in the excise duty on paper and elimination of all duties on stained paper in 1836 substantially lowered the price of wallpaper. A few years later, prices were further reduced by the introduction of machine-printed papers. The introduction of paper from wood pulp later in the century further decreased costs. The Victorian reverence for the concept of the home as a welcome refuge from a harsh outside world also encouraged the use of wallpaper because it gave Victorians, as Bartrip noted, "the opportunity to introduce colour, comfort and individuality into their rooms." British wallpaper production increased some thirtyfold between 1834 and 1874.[9]

Warnings against the possible dangers of arsenical wallpaper go back to at least 1839, when the German chemist Leopold Gmelin wrote in a letter to a newspaper that he had observed a mouse-like odor in rooms with such paper. He believed that the odor was due to a volatile arsenic compound that was potentially toxic. Reports of arsenic poisoning due to wallpaper soon began to appear in the literature. A British physician reported in 1851, for example, on the case of a young boy who had been poisoned as a result of chewing some green wallpaper containing arsenic. Another British medical practitioner, William Hinds, described in a medical journal in 1857 how some years earlier he had become ill with nausea and abdominal pains after redecorating a room with green wallpaper. Suspecting that the paper might be involved, he analyzed the pigment and found that it contained arsenic. After he removed the paper, his symptoms disappeared. Hinds had been motivated to publish his account eight years after the incident had occurred when he treated a couple for what he diagnosed as arsenic poisoning. The couple had recently had two rooms in their house covered with green wallpaper. Hinds believed that the problem was widespread. He argued that the pigment was loosely applied to the paper and that it could easily be rubbed off or dislodged in some other way as arsenic dust.[10]

Other physicians and scientists also began to criticize the use of arsenical wallpaper. Taylor testified about the arsenic content of wallpaper and its harmful effects before a parliamentary committee considering legislation to regulate the sale of poisons in 1857. Various cases of arsenic poisoning from wallpaper were reported in the medical literature. For example, in 1863 American physician William Rice described the case of a woman who had consulted him with symptoms of vomiting, abdominal pain, and weakness and trembling of the limbs. She explained to the doctor that her symptoms were always worse after sweeping and dusting her room. When Rice investigated the situation, he found that the walls of the woman's room "were covered with paper rich in green coloring matter, which I inferred to be Scheele's green." Upon testing the paper, he found that it did indeed contain arsenic, and he ordered the patient to either remove the paper or change residence.[11]

There was no question about the arsenic content of these papers, but there was disagreement as to whether or not the pigment posed a health hazard. There were those who disputed the concerns expressed by Taylor, Hinds, and others. Not surprisingly, the paper manufacturers argued for the safety of their products. One manufacturer announced that his rooms were covered in green paper and that he could rub it or lick it without dislodging the pigment. There were also some medical and scientific experts who questioned whether these papers were a threat to health. At the request of the British Board of Inland Revenue, a government chemist investigated the arsenical wallpapers that covered the walls of some of the rooms occupied by the Board. He concluded that the papers did not pose a threat to health. Arsenious acid, he argued, could not be vaporized at room temperature, so the only danger could come from arsenic dust brushed off unglazed papers. He believed that this problem could easily be managed by appropriate cleaning of the room. British physician Arthur Hill Hassall, a leader in the campaigns against food adulteration and against the use of arsenic pigment in artificial flowers, surprisingly defended arsenical wallpaper and fabric. He wrote to a scientific journal in 1859 that he himself owned green carpets, a green sofa and chairs, and several green table covers. He had examined various wallpapers and was convinced that the green pigments were too tightly bound to come loose from the paper (except in the case of some cheaply made papers), and he did not believe that any wallpaper was releasing arsenic into the air. He concluded that the chance of arsenic poisoning from such products was small.[12]

The most famous producer of wallpaper, the noted British designer and author William Morris, was also skeptical about the toxic effects of arsenic papers. Morris was one of the investors in the Devon Great Consols mine, the largest source of arsenic in the world. His design firm produced furniture, tapestries, wallpaper, metalware, glass, and a variety of other products. Wallpaper was one of the firm's staples. The evidence that many of Morris's papers contained arsenic is clear. Recently biologist Andrew Meharg investigated the Morris wallpapers. He obtained a sample from the William Morris Gallery of one of the designer's most famous papers, the Trellis pattern, and analyzed the green pigment. Meharg "showed unequivocally that the coloration was caused by a copper arsenic salt." He was also given access to a wallpaper sample book and with the aid of an X-ray fluorescence machine was able to show that nine of the first eleven papers designed by Morris contained arsenic.[13]

Morris expressed his doubts about the harmful effects of arsenic in his papers through his correspondence with his dye manufacturer. In response to a query from a worried customer, Mr. Nicholson, Morris dismissed the concerns of physicians and the public about arsenic poisoning from wallpaper, proclaiming, "As to the arsenic scare, a greater folly is hardly possible to imagine: the doctors were being bitten by witch fever." In a follow-up letter, he challenged the suggestion that the Nicholsons were poisoned by wallpaper: "For if they were a great number of people would be in the same plight and we should be sure to hear of it." One wonders if he became more sympathetic to the concerns of the consumer later in life, when he became a socialist and defender of the working class.[14]

Uncertainty about the mechanism by which arsenical wallpapers could poison residents of homes complicated the argument. Many people argued that only the poorest quality papers released arsenic dust into the air. On the other hand, it was known that the arsenic pigments did not vaporize at room temperature. So how could the poison exert its effect? Was it possible that a chemical reaction produced a toxic arsenic gas from the paper? Various experiments were carried out to test this hypothesis. For example, a room with arsenic wallpaper was tightly sealed for periods up to nine days, and the air in the room was then tested. No arsenic was detected in the air. The gas hypothesis would resurface and come to dominate later in the century, but attention focused at first more on the dust theory. Various investigators, such as Alfred Taylor, challenged the conclusions of Hassall and others that only cheaply made papers produced arsenic dust. There were numerous reports of the detection of fine arsenic dust on shelves and furnishings of rooms with arsenical wallpaper, even good quality paper. It was unclear, however, how much arsenic was actually breathed in by the inhabitants of the room and how much harm it did them. As Whorton has noted, the main evidence offered by physicians for the toxic effects of arsenic papers "was that illness disappeared when either the person or the paper was removed from the room."[15]

Although anxiety about arsenical wallpapers seems to have temporarily abated in the late 1860s, the subject attracted renewed attention in the following decade. The publication of a novel about the dangers of arsenical wallpaper, *The Green of the Period*, in 1869 may have helped to revive interest in the topic. In the 1870s articles in medical and public health journals kept the subject alive. A popular pamphlet by the British writer Henry Carr, *Our Domestic Poisons; or the Poisonous Effects of Certain Dyes and Colours Used in Domestic Fabrics* (1879), also highlighted the hazards posed by arsenic pigments in wallpaper and other products. Carr called for an end to the use of poisonous dyes in domestic products. In that same year, physician Jabez Hogg read a paper to the Royal Society of Medicine (RSM) of London in which he also called for prohibiting the sale of arsenical papers.

Hogg's paper led the RSM to establish a committee to investigate arsenic poisoning from wallpapers and other products. A questionnaire was sent to fifteen hundred physicians requesting information about relevant cases. The response rate was about 15 percent, and only fifty-four respondents provided detailed information on arsenic poisoning. Nevertheless, the committee recommended restrictions on the sale of arsenical products and a requirement that consumers be notified of the presence of the poison when such goods were sold. The committee also recommended that the subject be further investigated with the intent of accumulating additional evidence on the health hazards posed by arsenical products. Another British organization, the Royal Society of Arts (RSA), also initiated a study of the problem in 1880. The RSA, which was concerned with manufacturing, sent a questionnaire to businesses involved in the manufacture or application of colors. The full report of the committee was never published, but in its annual report for 1880 the RSA concluded that although the use of arsenical fabrics and papers had caused some illness and even death, "public dread" about the problem had been excessive. The report also suggested that the use of arsenic in such products was much less frequent than it had previously been or than was assumed. Critics argued that the RSA was too closely allied with trade and manufacture to view the subject impartially.

The subject was taken up in 1883 by the National Health Society (NHS), which hoped to provide an objective report. A subcommittee investigated the health hazards presented by arsenical products and recommended possible legislation on the matter. The subcommittee recommended a ban on the importation of arsenical wallpapers as a mechanism for countering domestic manufacturers' claims that if they stopped producing such papers, customers would simply switch to imported products. At the request of the subcommittee, the British government requested information from various foreign countries concerning legislation involving the production and sale of arsenic and other toxic pigments used to color wallpaper and textiles. At least seven of the countries to which queries were sent, including the United States, Belgium, Greece, and Italy, had no legislation in this area. The Germanic states had the most restrictive legislation. These findings challenged the views expressed by critics of arsenical products that Britain was far behind almost all other countries in regulating these products. In the end, Parliament took no action.[16]

Discussions of the dangers posed by arsenic pigments in wallpaper and other products also appeared in the medical literature and popular press in the United States in the period from about 1870.[17] In 1872 physician Frank Draper published an extensive overview of "the evil effects of the use of arsenic in certain green colors" in the *Annual Report of the State Board of Health of Massachusetts*. He reviewed the widespread use of arsenical colors in products such as artificial flowers, clothing, candy, toys, and paint. By far the largest portion of his report, however, was devoted to wallpaper. Draper stated:

> Important as are the topics which have thus far engaged our attention in the study of the arsenical greens and of the possible dangers incident to their use, they appear to have always been considered as of less significance than those relating to arsenical paper-hangings. . . . Distinguished scientific authorities in Germany, France, England and America have regarded the matter as one eminently deserving careful consideration, and the unanimity which characterizes the results of their studies can leave little room for doubt in unprejudiced minds concerning the harm which may ensue, under certain conditions, from the use of arseniferous wall-paper.[18]

Draper dismissed the "comparatively few" dissenters who questioned the harmful effects of such papers as either having based their experiments on false premises or as being biased in their conclusions. He also claimed that arsenical papers had declined in popularity some ten years earlier when their potential hazards were publicized, but he bemoaned the fact that the public seemed to have forgotten these warnings and that green papers had once again become fashionable (he did add that not all green papers contained arsenic). Draper's report included descriptions of a number of cases of arsenic poisoning from wallpaper. He rejected the kind of restrictive legislation enacted in some European countries as a way of treating the problem, noting that "such repressive legislation would be difficult in a society and under a government organized like our own." Instead, he optimistically looked to education of the public about these dangers as the means of eliminating the use of arsenical papers. Once people appreciated the hazards of arsenical papers, they would refuse to purchase them, "for reasonable people, informed concerning the risks, will not be likely to test their own tolerance of arsenic or to subject their children to it."[19]

Aware of Draper's report, Robert Kedzie of Michigan repeated Draper's warning about the dangers of arsenical wallpaper to the Michigan State Board of Health in the 1870s. Kedzie had obtained a medical degree from the University of Michigan in 1850. In 1863 he became professor of chemistry at the Michigan Agricultural College, the forerunner of Michigan State University, a position he held for the next thirty-nine years. Concerned about the destruction of Michigan's forests, Kedzie ran for and was elected to the Michigan House of Representatives in 1867. Determined to put science to use for the public good, he worked for conservation and consumer protection throughout his career. Kedzie also became actively involved in public health, serving on the Michigan Board of Health for eight years (the last four as president) from its founding in 1873. He also served as president of the American Public Health Association in 1882.

In the 1870s he investigated cases of otherwise healthy persons becoming mysteriously ill in a number of Michigan homes. The symptoms of those affected would disappear if they left the house or slept in another room. Suspecting the bright green wallpaper on the walls of these rooms, Kedzie subjected it to chemical analysis. He also analyzed the dust that had settled on the furniture. Kedzie demonstrated that the green pigment in the wallpaper was Paris green and that some of it came off the wallpaper as a fine dust that floated in the air of the room and coated the furniture.[20]

In addition to calling his Board of Health colleagues' attention to the toxic wallpaper, Kedzie also publicized the problem directly to the public. With the support of the Board of Health, he bought rolls of arsenical wallpaper from stores in three Michigan cities, cut up the paper, and bound samples in books to be distributed free to libraries around the state. He gave the book the melodramatic title *Shadows from the Walls of Death*. Kedzie also wrote an eight-page printed preface to the sample book, explaining the dangers of the deadly wallpaper (including descriptions of several reported cases of poisoning) and how to avoid them. He held the manufacturers of the papers responsible for the problem and called for "an enlightened public sentiment" to banish these papers from the home. Kedzie hoped that this book would "call attention to this source of danger, and to assist persons in detecting these dangerous colors in wall paper."[21]

The next major report on arsenic pigments in the United States was published in the 1880s by Edward S. Wood, professor of chemistry at Harvard Medical College. Wood's *Arsenic as A Domestic Poison* first appeared as a supplement in the 1884 report of the Massachusetts State Board of Health, Lunacy and Charity, but was then reprinted as a separate publication the following year. It was meant to be a follow-up to Draper's article in the report of the Massachusetts State Board of Health for 1872.[22]

Although Wood discussed arsenic pigments in a number of materials, such as articles of food and clothing, a substantial portion of the report is devoted to paper products. He saw wallpaper as a particularly serious problem, writing:

By far the most common source of domestic arsenical poisoning is wall-paper, which frequently contains an enormous amount of arsenic in the coloring matter. It was formerly supposed that the green papers were the only ones which were arsenical, but at the present time we find arsenic more frequently in wall-paper of other colors than green. This is probably due to the fact that the public has been more frequently informed in regard to the arsenical nature of green papers and pigments, and hence people are more liable to suspect the poisonous character of papers of this color, and to inquire of the dealer whether they are arsenical or not, than with regard to other colors.[23]

Wood was probably correct in assuming that by the 1880s, the public was becoming wary of green paper. As Bartrip has noted, the use of arsenical papers declined significantly in Britain in the late nineteenth century. Since no legislation was passed restricting its use in that country, Bartrip concluded that "consumer preference, stoked by adverse press publicity given to arsenically-coloured products, had encouraged change in commercial

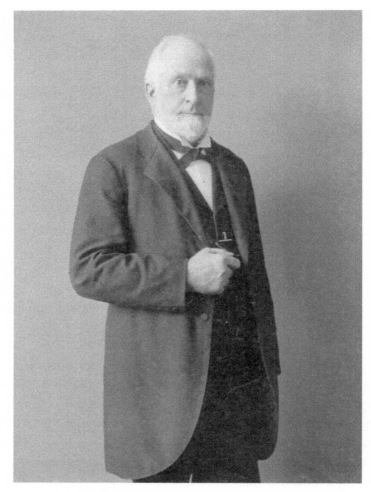

Robert Kedzie, a Michigan physician who campaigned for the elimination of arsenical wallpapers. *Courtesy of the Michigan State University Archives and Historical Collections.*

practice." Manufacturers found that consumers were reluctant to purchase products they knew were colored with arsenic pigments. In Britain, gaudy colors such as bright greens were also becoming less fashionable by this time.[24]

These same factors were at play in the United States, which also had no legislation restricting the manufacture or sale of arsenical wallpapers. Whorton has pointed out that there was a decline in the sale of arsenical wallpaper in the United States as well during this period. However, as Wood showed, arsenic pigments were still being used (at least in the United States) to dye papers colors other than green, where the consumer might not suspect the use of arsenic, as least well into the 1880s. In fact, publications in the 1890s and the early twentieth century continued to highlight the use of arsenic pigments in domestic products and they hazards that they presented. Even if all manufacture of arsenic wallpapers had ceased, however, there was still a problem with the large amounts of old papers that covered the walls of homes.[25]

As previously mentioned, the mechanism by which arsenic in wallpaper could poison individuals was unknown. Although early attempts to find arsenic dust in the air of papered rooms were not successful, by the 1850s house dust was shown to contain some arsenic. The manufacturers insisted that the arsenical pigments they used were permanently affixed to the paper. Those who supported the gas theory of arsenic poisoning argued that the problem could not be arsenic chips or dust coming off of the paper because people became ill in rooms where the arsenic wallpaper had been papered over with another arsenic-free layer. They suggested that some chemical reaction might result in the production of arsine or another toxic gas from the pigment on the wallpaper. There was speculation that a microorganism might be involved in the process.[26]

Finally in the 1890s an Italian physician, Bartolomeo Gosio, succeeded in isolating such a gas. As Cullen explained, "He exposed potato pulp containing 1 per cent arsenic trioxide to air and an intense garlic-like odor became apparent after the mixture became mouldy. He sucked the gas through a silver nitrate solution and then employed the Marsh test . . . to show that the solution contained arsenic. Gosio isolated pure moulds from the pulp and found that three of them were mainly responsible for the gas production."[27]

Gosio believed the gas was not arsine but probably an alkylarsenic derivative. He was able to show that he could produce this gas from arsenic pigments such as Scheele's green, as well as from arsenic trioxide. He even demonstrated that the gas could be produced by infecting an arsenical wallpaper with one of his gas-producing molds. Thus he had provided a possible mechanism by which an arsenic-containing gas could be generated from wallpaper. Gosio assumed the gas was toxic, but his experimental evidence was minimal and apparently flawed. For example, Cullen has recently criticized Gosio's experiments with rabbits, arguing that the animals probably died from pneumonia caused by spores produced by Gosio's mold rather than from the arsenical gas.[28]

It was widely assumed at the time, however, that Gosio gas, as the chemical came to be called, was the source of arsenic poisoning from wallpaper. Certain conditions, such as dampness, were believed to cause the growth of arsenic-producing molds on wallpaper. A 1904 publication from the U.S. Department of Agriculture noted that the work of Gosio and others had established "beyond doubt the fact that certain molds can set volatile compounds of arsenic free from fixed compounds of this element, which may be present in the wall paper or other materials in case a suitable medium for growth is present, such as the paste used in putting on wallpaper." As proof that this gas was toxic, the authors cited the numerous cases of illness among people living in rooms whose walls were covered with arsenical papers.[29]

Illness caused by arsenical wallpapers came to be called Gosio's disease. The 1931 deaths of two children in England from arsenic poisoning in which arsenical wallpapers were moldy stimulated Frederick Challenger and his colleagues at the University of Leeds to investigate the structure of Gosio gas. They established that the gas was trimethylarsine. Challenger accepted the view that this gas was toxic, and his work helped to reinforce and popularize this belief. Other research from as early as 1914 suggested that the compound Challenger identified as trimethylarsine was not very toxic, but these studies had little impact. In recent years, Cullen has challenged the belief that trimethylarsine is toxic. He has cited evidence to support his position and has suggested that the universal association of arsenic with poisoning contributed to the ease with which people readily accepted the idea of the toxicity of Gosio gas. The fact that arsine gas itself is highly toxic no doubt also played a role in the story.[30]

If Cullen is correct about the relative nontoxicity of trimethylarsine, then how does one account for the large number of reported cases of people who became ill while inhabiting rooms with arsenical wallpapers and then recovered when removed from those rooms? Cullen suggested that one possibility is that these individuals became sick from exposure to the mold itself rather than to any arsenical gas that it may have produced. We know that some molds produce mycotoxins that can cause illness, particularly in people with conditions such as asthma. Cullen also pointed out that nineteenth-century living conditions and public health standards were far from ideal. He concluded, "Illness attributed to arsenical wallpapers could have had many other causes. By about 1860 it had been realized that there was a serious problem with the widespread uses of arsenic and a reaction set in—arsenophobia ran wild in 19th century Europe and especially in Victorian England. An unseen and unknown poison gas, related to arsenic, could be used as a convenient excuse or scapegoat for mysterious, poorly understood illness."[31]

Arsenical wallpaper has figured in the controversy over the cause of death of Napoleon. The former emperor died in exile on the island of St. Helena in 1821. The official cause of death was given as cancer of the stomach, but from the beginning there was speculation about other possible causes. In the 1950s a theory was put forward that Napoleon was intentionally poisoned with arsenic after neutron activation of some samples of his hair were found to contain abnormal amounts of arsenic. David Jones and Kenneth Ledingham challenged this view in 1982, arguing that arsenic was used in so many products at the time that the emperor could have ingested it accidentally. They analyzed a sample of the wallpaper from the living room of Napoleon's residence on St. Helena and revealed that the paper contained arsenic. The paper had been hung in 1819, two years before Napoleon's death. The concentration of arsenic in the paper was relatively low by comparison with other papers of the day, and Jones and Ledingham concluded that it may have made Napoleon ill but probably did not kill him. The results of their analysis, however, prompted speculation that Napoleon had indeed died of arsenic poisoning, but that the poison had come from the wallpaper rather than from the hands of an assassin. Cullen has dismissed this theory as without foundation based on his investigation of Gosio gas.[32]

There is a clear-cut case of a notable person who became ill from a room containing arsenic, although the poison was in the paint rather than the wallpaper. Clare Boothe Luce, successful playwright and member of Congress, was appointed by President Dwight D. Eisenhower as ambassador to Italy in 1953. While living in Villa Taverna, the official residence of the United States ambassador, Luce became seriously ill. The cause was determined to be arsenic poisoning. The stucco roses on the ceiling of the room where she worked and slept were coated with a paint containing lead arsenate. Apparently vibrations from a washing machine on the floor above were shaking the ceiling and dislodging some of the paint, which created a constant film of arsenic-containing dust in the room.[33]

Arsenic in the Food Supply

Arsenic has been used as a poison to eliminate vermin such as rats for many centuries. The development of the German mining industry resulted in the availability of large quantities of white arsenic for the first time in Europe in the second half of the seventeenth century. This cheap, readily available substance was used from that time as a rat poison, the first effective poison widely available for this purpose. One historian has argued that the widespread use of arsenic as a rat poison may well have been a key factor in the disappearance of plague from Europe in this period.[34]

The introduction of arsenic to the food supply via pesticides, however, did not become a problem until arsenical pesticides became popular for the protection of crops from insects in the late nineteenth and early twentieth centuries. Paris green was the first of the arsenic insecticides, and it was introduced for this purpose in 1867. Within a relatively short time, it became popular with farmers, especially in the United States. Other arsenic compounds, such as London purple soon found their way on to the market as well. Lead arsenate was introduced in 1892, and by the early twentieth century it had become the most popular of all insecticides, a position that it was to hold until the introduction of dichlorodiphenyltrichloroethane (DDT) in World War II. Although more expensive than other arsenical insecticides, it was gentler to foliage and its success in halting the spread of the gypsy moth won it many converts.

In spite of their widespread use, arsenic pesticides had their critics. The potential dangers of arsenic poisoning to farmers, livestock, and possibly consumers were recognized. Nevertheless the effectiveness of these products in combating the pests that plagued farmers encouraged their use. As Whorton has written:

Arsenicals had detractors, and more than a few concerned farmers sympathized with the contributor to *Garden and Forest* who worried that "thousands of tons of a most virulent mineral poison in the hands of hundreds of thousands of people, to be freely used in fields, orchards and gardens all over the continent, will incur what in aggregate be a danger worthy of serious thought." In fact, much serious thought was given to the danger associated with the application of arsenic to corps, but while several distinct hazards were recognized, none was reckoned so serious as to proscribe the use of arsenicals.[35]

There was disagreement as to the threat posed to the consumer by residual arsenic on fruits and vegetables that reached the market. Supporters of the arsenicals often argued that the amounts were too small to be of consequence. Even those agricultural scientists who claimed that the residues were more substantial tended to believe that they did not pose a serious threat to health. Studies that seemed to indicate that even heavily sprayed crops were innocuous, however, overlooked the fact that these experiments were carried out under carefully controlled conditions, following the recommendations of entomologists (scientists who studied insects) on when and how much insecticide to spray. But farmers did not always follow these recommendations. They frequently sprayed too often, too heavily, or too close to the time that the crops would be harvested. Thus the amount of pesticide residues on many fruits and vegetables was probably higher than estimated on the basis of the controlled studies.[36]

As J. F. McDiarmid Clark has pointed out, concerns about arsenical insecticides were also muted by a focus in the medical profession on acute toxicity and a relative neglect of chronic toxicity. Spray residues were generally not present in large enough quantities on produce to cause acute arsenic poisoning. Repeated exposure to these levels of arsenic over time, however, could result in chronic poisoning, a fact that was often not sufficiently emphasized. It is always more difficult to demonstrate a cause and effect relationship when the effect may follow the cause only after many years.[37]

Britain was slower to adopt arsenic insecticides such as Paris green than the United States, largely because it did not have the same scale of insect devastation as America did. Many of the crops cultivated in North America in the nineteenth century were nonindigenous, and often new insect life accompanied these crops. With no native predators to keep them in check, these insects ran rampant. British entomologist Eleanor Ormerod, one of the few women in the field at the time, played a key role in promoting the use of Paris green in her native country after fruit growers turned to her in 1890 for advice on combating destructive caterpillars and moths. In February of 1891, she proudly proclaimed in a letter to a colleague: "Surely it should be recorded of me, 'SHE INTRODUCED PARIS-GREEN INTO ENGLAND.'"[38]

The use of arsenical insecticides in Britain was never comparable to that in America, but an incident in 1900 involving poisoned beer ultimately brought the safety issue to the attention of the British government. Physicians frequently encountered cases of peripheral neuritis in alcoholics in late-nineteenth-century Britain. In the fall of 1900, however, the number of cases reached epidemic proportions in the city of Manchester. About two thousand individuals were affected, and there were at least seventy deaths. Several signs pointed to the likelihood that something other than alcohol might be responsible for the large number of cases of neuritis. Although all the victims drank beer, some of them were only light to moderate drinkers, and certainly not alcoholics. In addition, the large majority of those afflicted came from the poorest classes and drank only cheap beer. Several physicians also noticed that the symptoms were more severe than in the usual cases of alcoholic neuritis. Was it possible that some toxic substance in cheap beer other than alcohol was responsible for the epidemic?

Several physicians detected small amounts of arsenic in cheap beer, and at least one of them concluded that the victims of the epidemic might be suffering from chronic arsenic poisoning. However, many doctors, who were used to treating patients with arsenical preparations, believed that the amount of arsenic in the beer was too small to poison those who drank it. Others suggested that perhaps the alcohol intensified the effect of the arsenic. The source of the arsenic was eventually traced to contaminated sulfuric acid that was used in the manufacture of glucose, which was commonly substituted for some of the malt in cheap beers. Removing the arsenic-contaminated beer from the market led to a drop in the incidence of peripheral neuritis in Manchester to pre-1900 levels, thus confirming the view that arsenic was indeed the culprit in the poisonings.

The Manchester beer incident led the British government to establish a Royal Commission to "Inquire into Arsenic Poisoning from the Consumption of Beer and Other Articles of Food and Drink" in 1901. The commission was chaired by one of Britain's most distinguished scientists, Lord Kelvin. Among the subjects discussed were the potential hazards of toxic spray residues on fruits and vegetables resulting from the use of arsenic pesticides. The commission recommended the setting of tolerance levels for arsenic in food and drink, proposing a limit for arsenic of .01 grains per gallon in liquids and .01 grains per pound in solids. The British government accepted these recommendations, and a number of other countries also adopted the commission's suggestions. With respect to pesticides, the amount of arsenic in spray residues on produce could thus not exceed .01 grains per pound.[39]

The United States did not set a tolerance for arsenical spray residues until the 1920s, prompted by pressure from abroad. European countries that imported American fruit began complaining as early as the 1890s about the excessive use of arsenical pesticides by American farmers. After the British tolerance had been set and came to be viewed essentially as a world tolerance, importers of American produce were further troubled by the fact that the United States had not adopted this standard. Finally, in 1925, matters came to a head when a British family became ill with arsenic poisoning that was traced to spray residues on apples imported from the Western United States. The British government seriously considered embargoing all American fruit, but the Department of Agriculture convinced the British to hold off on an embargo, promising to make every effort to see that fruit exported to Britain would meet the British arsenic tolerance. The British agreed to give the Americans a chance to remedy the situation before imposing an embargo.

Ironically, fruit designated for export thus began to receive greater scrutiny than fruit sold domestically. The Department of Agriculture's Bureau of Chemistry (BOC), predecessor of the Food and Drug Administration (FDA), decided to establish an informal and secret tolerance level for fruit for the domestic market, a tolerance that was more liberal than the British one. By the middle of 1926, however, the BOC decided that it needed to establish a stricter (and openly publicized) arsenic tolerance for domestic produce. For this purpose, it established a committee of experts to make a recommendation on the amounts of lead (the most commonly used pesticide by that time was lead arsenate) and arsenic that should be tolerated in food for human consumption. The committee, which held its first meeting on

January 3, 1927, was chaired by Reid Hunt, professor of pharmacology at Harvard University, and consisted of a number of distinguished scientists. Hunt's committee recommended an arsenic tolerance of .021 grains per pound, about twice the British tolerance. Surprisingly, the BOC, after establishing the Hunt Committee, chose to ignore its recommendations and instead accept the stricter British tolerance. A possible explanation for this decision is that accepting the lower arsenic level would also better control the lead residue. Lead analysis at the time was a slow and tedious process, and thus it was quicker and easier to control the lead residue indirectly through the arsenic residue.[40]

Although the arsenic pesticides were largely replaced by DDT and other compounds after World War II, they did not entirely disappear from the agricultural scene. The more toxic inorganic arsenic compounds, such as lead arsenate, were largely abandoned, although they continued to find some use for special purposes, such as measles (a fungus infection) in grapes. Several less toxic organic arsenic compounds continue to be used as herbicides and fungicides up to the present time. For example, monomethylarsonic acid is almost universally used to control weeds on golf courses. This compound breaks down into inorganic arsenic, which can leach into groundwater, and it can also move through wildlife food chains, leading to concerns about potential damaging effects on human and animal health. In 2009 the U.S. Environmental Protection Agency reached a voluntary agreement with users of these products to phase them out over a period of four years.[41]

Pesticides, however, were not the only means of introducing arsenic into the food supply. As previously noted, arsenical dyes were used to color many products, including some foodstuffs such as candy and other sweets. Articles published in *The Lancet* reported as early as the 1830s on the common use of arsenic pigments to provide the green color in confectionary. Cases of arsenical poisoning of children from eating sweets such as cake decorations appeared in the medical literature in Britain in the 1840s and 1850s. Arthur Hill Hassall, the prominent British physician who was a pioneer in the study of food adulteration, published his studies on colored confectionary in 1854. He found that more than a dozen toxic substances were used to color sweets, including arsenic. In the United States, the humor magazine *Puck* complained about the use of arsenic greens in confectionary in 1885, referring to "fiends who are said to have used poison in the construction of candy." Green confectionery came to be so feared that as late as the 1950s it was still difficult to sell green confections in many parts of Scotland.[42]

The most serious individual incident involving arsenic-poisoned candies, however, did not involve the intentional use of this poison, although it was a case of food adulteration. It was common in mid-nineteenth century Britain for confectioners to use an inert substance referred to as "daft" (probably mostly plaster of Paris) to replace some of the considerably more expensive sugar in their products. In 1858 a sweetmaker named Joseph Neal in the city of Bradford made a batch of peppermint candies using daft that he had obtained from a local pharmacist. Unfortunately, the pharmacist's assistant who provided the product mistook white arsenic for the daft. By the time the authorities had traced the source of the problem and removed the remaining sweets from the market, about two hundred people had become ill, and some twenty had died as a result of consuming the candy. Although no one was convicted of any crime in connection with the Bradford poisonings, the incident did play a role in the passage of the Act for Preventing the Adulteration of Articles of Food and Drink of 1860 and the Pharmacy Act of 1868. Unfortunately, the former law was too weak and lenient to have much effect on adulteration, and Hassall reported in 1876 that arsenical pigments were still being used to color confectionery. A food and drug bill passed the previous year, however, was beginning to provide more rigorous regulation of the marketplace. Among the provisions of the Pharmacy Act was a requirement that the sale of poisons be restricted to qualified pharmacists.[43]

James Whorton has described another example of arsenic in the food supply, this time involving the adulteration of wine, that had begun by the eighteenth century. Wines were commonly treated at the time with isinglass, a form of collagen obtained from the dried swim bladders of fish, in order to "fine," or clarify, them. Those responsible for the fining process, however, discovered that arsenic worked just as well and was significantly cheaper. The color of red wines was dulled by the arsenic, but white wines were actually given a desirable gloss by the metal. In the late 1700s, as much as five hundred pounds of arsenic was being used annually in London for the fining of white wines. There were reports of arsenic poisoning from white wine resulting in illness or death as early as the 1720s.[44]

In spite of enormous advances in science and in the regulation of food and drugs, concerns are still expressed today about the possible hazards of arsenic in the food supply. Arsenic occurs in the environment both naturally and as a result of contamination from past and present use of products containing the metal (e.g., pesticides, herbicides, and wood preservatives). Arsenic can thus find its way into the soil and water and possibly contaminate food products as well as drinking water supplies. Food can also be contaminated during manufacturing or processing. In 2009 the European Food Safety Authority's Panel on Contamination in the Food Chain issued a report on arsenic in food. The panel noted that conclusions about the health effects of arsenic in food were hindered by the fact that most studies analyzing arsenic content did not distinguish between organic and inorganic arsenic. Arsenic bound in organic compounds tends to be much less toxic than arsenic in the form of inorganic compounds such as arsenic trioxide. Based on available data and making a number of assumptions, the panel concluded that some consumers were at risk of chronic arsenic poisoning. They specifically identified frequent consumers of rice and algae-based products. They also identified children as possibly being at greater risk.[45]

Another area of current concern involves the addition of arsenic to the food of chickens in order to promote growth, kill parasites, and improve the pigmentation of the meat. This practice appears to have grown out of work in the 1930s that identified copper arsenite as the active ingredient in medication given to poultry in their drinking water to control coccidiosis, a disease of chickens. Other inorganic arsenic compounds were then tested, but all were found too toxic for practical use. Aware of the use of certain organic arsenic compounds in medicine, researchers began to investigate these substances and found that roxarsone (3-nitro-4- hydroxyphenylarsonic acid) was the most effective drug against coccidiosis. By chance, it also turned out that this compound stimulated growth in chickens. By the 1940s, organic arsenicals were being added to chicken feed. In the United States, about 2.2 million pounds of roxarsone (by far the most common arsenic-based additive) are mixed with chicken feed each year. Although roxarsone is a relatively low-toxicity organic arsenic compound, some of the additive is converted into more toxic inorganic arsenic in the body of the chicken. The result is that some inorganic arsenic gets into the chicken meat and eggs. In addition, chicken excrement containing arsenic is used as a fertilizer for crops, lawns, and gardens, leading to increased amounts of arsenic in soil, groundwater, and ultimately drinking water.

Worries about arsenic poisoning led the European Union to ban arsenic additives in 1999. In 2004 Tyson Foods, the largest poultry producer in the United States, discontinued their use. Another major American poultry producer, Perdue, has also abandoned the use of arsenic in chicken feed. The restaurant chain McDonald's has also asked its suppliers not to use arsenic additives. Yet arsenic is still being added to chicken feed on some poultry farms today, although there have been ongoing efforts to eliminate this practice. The Maryland legislature, for example, introduced a bill to ban arsenic in chicken feed in 2011, although it was defeated by opposition from poultry farmers.[46]

Although about 90 percent of roxarsone's use is in chickens, it is also used to a more limited extent in turkey and swine feed in the United States, China, and other countries. One study by Canadian veterinarians reported cases on two different farms of severe arsenic poisoning in young pigs that ingested feed containing roxarsone. In the case of swine, the margin of safety between the recommended dose and the toxic dose is small. As in the case of chickens, arsenicals also find their way into pig manure, causing contamination of soil when this manure is used as fertilizer. In the midst of this controversy over arsenic in animal feed, the manufacturer of roxarsone, Pfizer, announced in June 2011 that it was going to suspend sale of the drug in thirty days while it does a "full scientific assessment" of the drug, a move cheered by consumer advocates.[47]

A study of baby foods by Swedish scientists in 2011 has raised additional concerns about arsenic in foods. The investigators tested products of major baby food manufacturers and found that feeding infants twice a day on baby foods such as rice porridge could increase their exposure to arsenic by up to fifty times when compared to breastfeeding alone. Arsenic levels were especially high in rice-based foods. The study prompted calls for new restrictions on arsenic and other toxic elements in food.[48]

By far the most serious problem of ingestion of arsenic today, however, involves drinking water.

Arsenic in Drinking Water

Concerns about arsenic in drinking water go back to at least the nineteenth century. In the 1840s, for example, boys at a military academy near Vienna became ill, and some died, before it was discovered that the source of the problem was a well. The well was found to contain the remains of rats that had been exterminated with arsenic, which was assumed to be responsible for the poisoning of the students. Warnings were issued to the public about using arsenic to kill rats on premises containing wells, but arsenic continued to be commonly used as a rat poison. Whorton claims that there do not appear to be any authenticated cases of arsenic poisoning from dead rats in well water. However, well water has been contaminated by arsenic from industry. In one case, people in the neighborhood of a manufacturer of colored paper were poisoned over a period of thirty years before it was discovered that the cause was arsenic from the factory that had seeped into the groundwater. Arsenic from smelters also sometimes found its way into springs and other sources of drinking water, as in the city of Reichenstein in the late nineteenth century.[49]

These examples were localized and isolated incidents, but in recent times arsenic poisoning from drinking water has become a massive and widespread problem in Bangladesh and in the Indian state of West Bengal. Ironically, this problem was caused by an effort to save lives and improve health. In the 1970s almost a quarter of a million people were dying in Bangladesh alone from waterborne diseases because of drinking water supplies contaminated with pathogenic microorganisms. A possible solution appeared to be tapping the huge repository of pure water coming from the Himalayas in the sediments being swept onto the Bengal plain. This water could be obtained through the use of cheap tube well technology, involving pushing iron tubes through the soft sediment and fitting the tops of the tubes with a hand pump to bring water to the surface. Although tube wells have been used to a limited extent in Bangladesh since the 1930s, it was not until the 1970s that the rate of construction became significant. The United Nations Children's Fund (UNICEF) began a massive campaign in 1972 that involved the construction of close to a million tube wells throughout Bangaldesh. The governments of Bangladesh and West Bengal, with the help of international aid agencies, sank many more such wells, and many citizens and communities did the same. By 2000 there were probably close to 11 million tube wells in these areas, and about 97 percent of the rural population of Bangladesh drew its drinking water from them.

The immediate health benefits of the tube wells soon became obvious. Infant mortality was cut in half, and the mortality rate of children under the age of five dropped from 247 per 1,000 to 112 per 1,000 over the period from 1960 to 1996. But the tube wells introduced an unexpected health problem. In 1983 Dr. K. C. Saha, a dermatologist at the Calcutta School of Tropical Medicine, made the first diagnosis of a person with arsenical dermatosis resulting from drinking arsenic-rich tube well water. This was only the first of 1,214 cases from sixty-one separate villages that he identified over the next four years. Saha described the hyperpigmentation (a black raindrop pattern on the limbs, chest and back) that resulted from the arsenicosis and reported some cases of skin cancer among these patients. He also determined that the arsenic content of their drinking water was excessively high. This discovery was not welcome news, and Saha almost lost his job as a result of reporting these findings. The government of West Bengal did little to address the well water situation.

Other Calcutta-based scientists published articles calling attention to the problem in 1988 and in 1993, but aid agency and government officials apparently could not, or would not, believe what they were hearing. The governments of Bangladesh and West Bengal, and the world at large, have been slow to respond to this crisis. The health benefits of the tube wells, in terms of illness and death due to infectious disease, were so great that it was difficult to believe that people were also becoming ill from this water. Arsenic-related diseases did not begin to show up in patients until after about ten years of drinking the tube well water, and so the magnitude of the problem was not immediately apparent. The digging of tube wells continued at a prodigious pace throughout the 1990s.

Scottish scientist Andrew Meharg has summarized the situation: "The puncturing of the Earth's skin with tens of millions of wells has drawn out poison—not just any poison, but the most notorious of all: arsenic. Over one hundred million people may now be at risk of routinely drinking dangerous levels of arsenic, an element that causes skin, bladder and lung cancer, stillbirths and heart attacks."

The subtitle of Meharg's book, *Venomous Earth*, calls the problem of arsenic in drinking water "the world's worst mass poisoning." Although Bangladesh and West Bengal have received the most publicity, arsenic in drinking water is affecting citizens in numerous countries in Asia, Africa, Europe, and North and South America. Estimates of the number of people being poisoned by arsenic in their drinking water range from a conservative 140 million in 70 countries to a staggering 500 million or more. Whatever the exact number, it is certainly very large and a matter of great concern. Efforts are underway in various countries to mitigate the problem, but solutions can be slow and expensive. Arsenic-mitigation methods include digging very deep tube wells (down to water that is generally arsenic-free), harvesting rainwater, and using surface water that has been treated to eliminate pathogenic microorganisms.[50]

Arsenic and Beauty

Unlike other toxic metals, such as lead, arsenic does not appear to have found significant use for cosmetic purposes throughout much of history. In the nineteenth century, however, the use of arsenic to help produce a fair complexion became common in Europe and America. A major reason for this trend appears to have been the growing awareness of arsenic eaters in Styria.[51]

Although arsenic eating in Styria may go back to the sixteenth or seventeenth century, it did not receive much attention in the rest of Europe until the nineteenth century, when a number of reports on the practice appeared in the medical and popular literature. With respect to its cosmetic use by women, American chemist James F. Johnston gave the following romanticized account in his popular 1855 book on *The Chemistry of Common Life*:

> But the Styrian peasant-girl, stirred by an unconsciously growing attachment—confiding scarcely to herself her feelings, and taking counsel of her inherited wisdom only—really adds, by the use of hidri, to the natural graces of her filling and rounding form, paints with brighter hues her blushing cheeks and tempting lips, and imparts a new and winning lustre to her sparkling eye. Everyone sees and admires the reality of her growing beauty: the young men sound her praises, and

become suppliants for her favour. She triumphs over the affections of all, and compels the chosen one to her feet.

Thus even cruel arsenic, so often the minister of crime and the parent of sorrow, bears a blessed jewel in its forehead, and, as a love-awakener, becomes at times the harbinger of happiness, the soother of ardent longings, the bestower of contentment and peace![52]

What woman could resist such an appeal? Reports of the "clear and blooming complexions" and full rounded figures of the young Styrian peasant women led to widespread use of arsenic as a cosmetic in many countries. The arsenic was taken in various forms—women often drank Fowler's solution, a popular arsenical medicine, or used it as a cosmetic wash. Some actually used white arsenic as a hair powder, perhaps to kill vermin. Sulphide of Arsenicum was advertised as a skin remedy and "the sure way to a better complexion." Products such as Dr. Simms Arsenic Complexion Wafers were popular, as were arsenical soaps. In general, however, these arsenical wafers and soaps contained very little arsenic.[53]

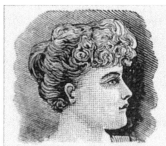

LADIES

If you desire a transparent, CLEAR, FRESH complexion, free from blotch, blemish, roughness, coarseness, redness, freckles, or pimples, use

DR. CAMPBELL'S
SAFE ARSENIC COMPLEXION WAFERS
—— AND ——
Fould's Medicated Arsenic Complexion Soap.

The only real true beautifiers in the world. *Warranted to give satisfaction* in every case or money refunded. Wafers by mail, $1 ; six large boxes, $5. Soap, per cake, 50 cents.

Address, H. B. FOULD, 214 Sixth Avenue, New York.
SOLD BY DRUGGISTS EVERYWHERE.

An advertisement for Dr. Campbell's Safe Arsenic Complexion Wafers, 1896.
Courtesy of Period Paper.

Arsenic-based cosmetics were still on the American market at least as late as the 1930s. The 1933 muckraking book *100,000,000 Guinea Pigs*, which called for stricter regulation of foods, drugs and cosmetics, cited several examples. The authors identified and attacked, for example, a number of hair tonics that contained arsenic. They were especially critical of a product called Dr. James P. Campbell's Safe Arsenic Complexion Wafers, arguing that putting the word "safe" before "arsenic" in no way diminished the toxicity of the product. This product was intended not only for improving complexion, but was advertised as a cure for numerous diseases, including cancer of the lip and womb, malaria, diabetes, tuberculosis, and snake bites.[54]

It is impossible to know how many people were harmed by these arsenic cosmetics. Some of the products contained relatively little arsenic and were probably harmless. Other preparations contained larger quantities of arsenic and could have resulted in poisoning, especially if the dose employed were high or the use of the product prolonged. For example, Catherine Bennett, known as the most beautiful woman in St. Louis, apparently died of arsenic poisoning in 1859 as the result of extensive cosmetic use of arsenic.[55] Many people certainly viewed the practice as dangerous, as evidenced by the criticism expressed in *100,000,000 Guinea Pigs*.

There were critics of the cosmetic use of arsenic in the nineteenth century as well. For example, the American humor magazine *Punch* discussed in 1869 the new mania of New York women eating arsenic in order to achieve brilliant complexions. *Punch* called this habit a form of "fashionable" insanity or suicide that prompted women to poison their bodies in order to improve their appearance.[56] Such notables as the dancer Lola Montez and Catherine Beecher, pioneer in the cause of women's education, spoke out against the use of arsenic as a beauty aid, as did a number of women's magazines and medical publications. One book by two physicians even suggested that women who consume arsenic no doubt exhaled enough of the poison to render them undesirable as wives.[57] This claim appears to be reminiscent of the legend of the "poison maiden," found in the literature of India and other cultures. The poison maiden was a woman who was supposedly transformed into a vial of poison after consuming small amounts of toxic substances over many years. She could then be used as a weapon to eliminate one's enemies by seducing them and killing them with her deadly kisses and breath. One story, for example, tells how Aristotle saved

Alexander the Great's life by warning him about a poison maiden who was given to him as a gift by another monarch. This legend was apparently the stimulus for Nathaniel Hawthorne's short story "Rappaccini's Daughter," in which a young woman becomes toxic to all she touches through years of exposure to the poisonous plants produced by her physician-father's experiments.[58]

Toxic Wood

Because wood is a source of food for organisms such as fungi and insects, efforts to preserve it by the use of various substances (e.g., pitch, olive oil) go back to ancient times. By the eighteenth century, chemicals such as copper sulfate and mercuric chloride were being used as wood preservatives. In 1838 two substances that were widely adopted for wood preservation were patented in England. John Bethel obtained a patent for the use of creosote, which he injected into wood under pressure. William Burnett patented the use of zinc chloride for the preservation of wood. These substances all had their disadvantages. Creosote, a derivative of coal tar, was a complex mixture that could vary in chemical composition and physical properties. It could not be painted, had an odor, and sometimes bled. Mineral salts such as zinc chloride were easily washed out of the wood, could corrode and reduce the strength of wood, and decreased electrical resistance.

By the 1920s sodium dichromate was being added to copper sulfate. This process resulted in the formation of chromium-lignin complexes and the production of stable copper chromate, helping prevent the copper from being leached out of the wood. Another problem with copper sulfate, however, was that many fungi, especially brown rot, can tolerate copper. Because of its known pesticide and preservative properties, arsenic was also sometimes used to protect wood; oak fence posts were sometimes preserved by filling holes drilled in the wood below the ground surface with arsenic trioxide. Karl Wolman experimented with various chemicals and processes for wood preservation, including arsenic, in the first few decades of the twentieth century and has generally been credited with introducing the modern process of pressure-treating wood.

The wood preservative that eventually came to dominate the market, known as chromated copper arsenate (CCA), was introduced by an Indian mining engineer in 1933. Sonti Kamesan, working in the Wood Preservation

Section of the Forest Research Institute Dehradun, was trying to find a more effective preservation for the timber used as supports in mines. Rotting timbers that collapsed in mines were a major safety risk. Kamesan used a combination of arsenic and copper, which was effective against insects and fungi, and added chromium to the formula to bind the two toxins to the wood fibers. He patented CCA, which was marketed under the name Ascu. The compound was popularized in the United States in part through its use by the Bell Telephone Company for the preservation of telephone poles.[59]

Some woods such as cedar and pine are naturally resistant to rotting caused by insects and fungi, but supplies of these woods decreased beginning in the 1970s. The search for an inexpensive replacement led to the extensive use of cheaper wood such as pine and fir impregnated with CCA. This wood is often referred to as pressure-treated wood because the chemicals are forced into the cells under high pressure. Treated wood became popular as it proved resistant to most pests and was relatively inexpensive. According to the EPA, about 70 percent of single family homes in the United States have decks or porches made of CCA-treated wood, and many public playgrounds also have CCA-treated wood structures. As of 1990, about 90 percent of the arsenic produced worldwide was being used for wood preservation.

In the 1980s concerns about the safety of CCA-treated wood increased. The EPA released a study in 1986 claiming that CCA-treated wood was safe to handle. Since the EPA was in the process of reviewing and eventually banning the use of arsenic pesticides, some members of the public viewed this report with skepticism. The Consumer Product Safety Commission (CPSC), influenced by industry pressure, shelved a proposal that the wood carry a warning label and developed instead a set of voluntary and weak guidelines. The industry continued to argue that CCA-treated wood was perfectly safe. But a number of publicized incidents and jury verdicts in favor of persons claiming they had been poisoned by the wood damaged the credibility of the industry. Cullen described one such case: "Jimmy Sipes worked for the U.S. Forest Service in Indiana where he occasionally sawed wood to make picnic tables. In 1983 after 10 days of sawing he began to vomit blood. He recovered slowly but had a relapse after another stint with the saw. In the hospital he was found to have about 100 times the normal concentration of arsenic in his hair and finger nails. A jury awarded him $100,000."[60]

In 2001 the subject made headlines when two Florida newspapers ran a series of articles about arsenic leaching out of CCA-treated wood structures. Florida officials found elevated levels of arsenic in the soil under pressure-treated wood playground equipment and closed a number of parks. At about the same time, several scientific studies were issued that demonstrated that arsenic and chromium do leach out of CCA-treated wood into the soil and on to the surface of the structures. Interested groups petitioned the CPSC to ban the use of CCA-treated wood in playground equipment and to assess the safety of the product in general.

These events prompted the EPA to review its Consumer Awareness Program and the guidelines concerning arsenic-treated wood. Eventually, the agency included in its guidelines the recommendation that CCA-treated wood contain statements that the wood contains arsenic and that some of the preservative chemicals might migrate into the soil or become dislodged from the wood upon contact with skin. The guidelines remained voluntary, however, and thus essentially unenforceable. Continued controversy and pressure prompted the EPA and the industry to reach a voluntary agreement in 2002 to eliminate the use of CCA-treated wood for consumer use by December 31, 2003. The manufacturers of CCA also agreed to gradually reduce their production of the preservative to give wood treatment plants time to switch to arsenic-free preservatives. CCA is still used for treating such products as utility poles and marine timbers. In 2002 the European Union announced a ban on the use of arsenic as a wood preservative although continuing to allow it for limited uses such as telephone poles and railroad ties.

Although the production of arsenic-preserved wood for consumer use has now ended, there are still numerous wooden structures in homes and playgrounds that contain the chemical. The EPA has indicated that it does not believe that these structures pose any unreasonable risk to the public, a position echoed by the industry. Many members of the public are not convinced that CCA-treated wood is generally safe, especially for use in children's playgrounds. Many local authorities have chosen to replace such playground equipment with structures made of metal or other arsenic-free materials. Various coatings have also been applied to treated wood structures to reduce the leaching of the preservative chemicals. A recent study from the University of California, San Francisco, concluded that CCA residues are not easily absorbed through the skin, but this report is not likely to quell all concerns about CCA-treated wood, especially on the part of parents.

Concerns about the safest method for disposing of all of CCA-treated wood from countless structures around the country have also surfaced. Incinerating the wood leaves a residue of ash containing arsenic, and dumping it in a landfill results in the arsenic leaching into the soil over time. The EPA has recommended, but not required, that CCA-treated wood be disposed of in lined landfills so that the effluent can be collected for treatment. The debris from Hurricane Katrina in 2005 is estimated to contain 1,740 tons of arsenic, which could eventually leach into the environment, since it was disposed of in an unlined landfill.[61]

Arsenic in the Atmosphere

Arsenic compounds enter the atmosphere from both natural sources, such as volcanoes, and human activities, such as smelting of ores and burning of fossil fuels. Arsenic in the atmosphere is predominantly absorbed on particulate matter and is usually present in inorganic forms. In general, the level of arsenic in the air is not sufficient to cause health problems, but higher levels can accumulate in localized areas where large amounts of arsenic compounds are released into the atmosphere.

Coal and oil shale contain higher concentrations of arsenic and certain other metals than petroleum. Increased use of these fuels has thus led to increased release of arsenic into the atmosphere, although some processes that have been introduced, such as washing coal to remove sulfur before burning, removes some of the arsenic. According to a study conducted by the Oak Ridge National Laboratory in the 1970s, the consumption of coal by power plants released about 3,000 tons of arsenic into the atmosphere at that time. However, power plants are widely disbursed across the country, and so the concentration of arsenic in the air surrounding any individual power plant may not be enough to produce harmful effects.[62]

Concern about arsenic in the atmosphere has largely centered upon smelters, especially copper smelters, and the environments in their vicinity. One of the most famous of the incidents of arsenic poisoning from smelters involved the Anaconda Copper Mining Company's (ACMC) smelting facilities in Deer Lodge Valley, Montana, in the early twentieth century.

The city of Butte, Montana, emerged as a major copper-mining center in the 1880s, and a number of new companies built smelters in the area. These new facilities placed a heavy burden on the water and timber resources of the Butte region and also resulted in heavy air pollution in the city. Timothy LeCain has described the extent of the pollution problem: "During the late nineteenth century, the pollution from Butte copper-smelting operation had sometimes been so thick that workers reportedly lost their way while walking home, and carriage drivers were required to hire a man with a lantern to warn pedestrians of their approach. Worse, the smoke caused or aggravated all manner of lung diseases. Death rates from pneumonia and tuberculosis soared, exceeding the tolls in even highly urbanized cities such as Chicago and London."[63]

The largest and most important of these copper companies was the ACMC. After unsuccessful efforts to reduce its pollution, the company decided in 1883–1884 to build a smelting facility in rural Deer Lodge Valley, about twenty-six miles west of Butte, a site that provided them with ample water and timber and where there were many fewer people to complain about the pollution. By 1902 ACMC had opened three smelters in the Deer Valley Lodge area.

The problems with local farmers and ranchers began with the opening of the largest of these smelters, the Washoe complex, in 1902. This facility processed about seven thousand tons of ore a day, belching forth huge quantities of gases in the process. Although the plant was modern and increased production, the company had done nothing to reduce pollution. Within months of the opening of the smelter, farmers and ranchers in the valley began to complain of unusually high deaths of livestock, and they were convinced that the new smelter was to blame for these deaths. State veterinarians performed autopsies on the animals and determined that they had ingested deadly amounts of arsenic, one of the constituents of the smelter smoke. As LeCain noted, "The new location, in concert with the Washoe complex's tremendously increased rate of production, meant that the winds were now scattering some twenty tons of arsenic over the farms of Deer Valley Lodge every day, a figure that shot up to as much as seventy-five tons a day during the wartime boom of 1918."[64]

After paying more than $330,000 in claims to farmers in order to settle these complaints, the company temporarily shut down the facility in 1903 in order to avoid further liability. ACMC built a new three-hundred-foot smokestack and added dust chambers designed to settle out the arsenic particles in an effort to deal with the pollution problem and reopened the smelter. But the deaths of livestock continued, and a group of farmers and ranchers entered into a lengthy legal battle with the company. At the same time, farmers in other states were also taking the smelting industry to court. In 1904 they won a significant victory when federal district judge John A. Marshall ruled against the smelter owners in Salt Lake City, effectively shutting down the Salt Lake smelter industry. The Deer Lodge Valley Farmers' Association was greatly encouraged by this decision.

The Deer Lodge Valley group was to be disappointed, however. After a trial lasting four years and involving 237 witnesses, federal judge William H. Hunt ruled in favor of ACMC. As Fredric Quivik explained, "Judge Hunt ruled that there did appear to be arsenical poisoning in the Deer Lodge Valley. Nevertheless, he held in favor of the ACMC because of what he considered the more important argument: the economic damage done to the Butte and Anaconda areas if the smelter were to close would be greater than the damage that the smelter smoke might be causing the farmers."[65]

The issue of possible harm to humans in the area does not seem to have played a role in the trial or decision. The farmers appealed their case all the way up to the Supreme Court, but they lost at every step. Under pressure from the federal government, the ACMC agreed to the formation of a board of experts, the Anaconda Smoke Commission, which would investigate the problem and make recommendations for its resolution, which the firm agreed to follow. This process also dragged on, and the company continued to resist efforts to invest in better pollution control. Finally, in 1919, they did make changes recommended by the commission, but tests revealed that over half the arsenic was still escaping into the atmosphere. It was not until 1923 that the company added equipment that removed most of the arsenic from the smelter. Even then, the arsenic output was about twenty-five tons per day, about one-third of its wartime level and similar to earlier levels. At this point, the commission decided that the arsenic output was no longer a nuisance to the surrounding community and declared the problem solved.

Ironically, the arsenic removed from the smelter smoke was essentially fed back into the environment in the form of pesticides and arsenic-treated wood.[66]

Another major company involved in arsenic production is Asarco, a subsidiary of the Mexican firm Grupo Mexico SA. Asarco operated a lead and arsenic smelter in Everett, Washington, from 1894 to 1912. Significant amounts of arsenic were released into the air, although the company did try to trap as much of the arsenic trioxide as they could for sale. Asarco became the world's largest arsenic producer. The production of arsenic was later moved to other locations, eventually winding up in Tacoma, Washington. The arsenic concentration in the air at the worksite was high, increasing the risk of respiratory cancer death. Residents of communities near this and other smelters were also concerned about their health. Asarco funded studies in the 1980s and 1990s that concluded that there was little risk of lung cancer mortality due to smelter emissions, but some were skeptical of these results. As regulations and standards were tightened, arsenic trioxide production became less attractive, and the company abandoned production of the chemical in 1985. Long after smelting activities have ceased at a site, however, the area may remain contaminated with arsenic and other toxic substances. With respect to Asarco, Cullen has reported, "The company has been found liable for contaminating 94 sites in 24 US states. The sites, some entire towns, include some of the largest Superfund areas. . . . The cost of the cleanup is estimated to be well over $1 billion (US)."[67]

Arsenic is ubiquitous in the environment, and comes from both natural sources and as the result of human activity. Arsenic in the environment may occur in the land, air, or water. Beginning in the nineteenth century, arsenic was used for a wide variety of industrial and commercial purposes, perhaps most notably as a green pigment for wallpaper, paint, fabrics, and a host of other products. Although its use as a pigment decreased dramatically in the twentieth century, other uses of the chemical, such as in pesticides and as wood preservatives, were initiated or increased significantly. In recent decades, there have been substantial efforts to replace arsenic for most purposes. We are still confronted, however, with problems of arsenic in the environment, the most serious of which is arsenic in drinking water in various parts of the world. Some scientists, however, believe that the threat posed by arsenic in the environment has been exaggerated, and speak of "arseno-phobia," an irrational fear of the chemical based on its traditional reputation as a poison. On the whole, however, most scientific and medical authorities seem to be convinced of the potential dangers of exposure to arsenic in various products and environments, including the possibility of cancers caused by long-term exposure.[68]

CHAPTER FIVE

What Kills Can Cure
Arsenic in Medicine

It may seem odd that the substance thought of as the quintessential poison has also had a long history of use as a medicine. Yet arsenic compounds have been employed as remedies in various illnesses from antiquity up to the present time. This fact is not as surprising as it might at first seem. After all, almost all medicines, even those developed in recent times, have toxic side effects, sometimes serious ones. In the sixteenth century, Paracelsus pointed out that all things are poisons in the right doses. Too much of a seemingly innocuous substance such as salt, for example, can be lethal. When Paracelsus was criticized for recommending the use of dangerous chemicals such as salts of arsenic, mercury, and lead in the treatment of disease, he responded that these substances could indeed be beneficial if administered in small, controlled doses. The difference between a medicine and a poison was a question of amount or dose.[1]

Paracelsus was not the first physician to employ arsenic for medicinal purposes, however. The earliest use of arsenic as a remedy goes back to ancient times and is lost to history. It was not used in its elemental form, but as one of its salts. One of the earliest references to arsenic in medicine appears in the writings attributed to the Greek physician Hippocrates (ca. 460–360 BC), often called the father of medicine. Hippocrates recommended the use of realgar and orpiment in the treatment of ulcers (sores) on the body, as did the noted Greco-Roman physician Galen in the second century AD. In his famous treatise on materia medica (medicine or drugs), Dioscorides (first century AD), aware of the astringent and corrosive properties of orpiment, advocated its use as a depilatory (hair remover). He also recommended realgar mixed with oil to destroy lice, as well as the inhalation of its vapors for chronic cough. The use of arsenic as a medicine has a long tradition in the East as well. The ancient Chinese were using orpiment and realgar to treat abscesses and skin diseases by 200 BC. Reportedly, arsenic compounds were also used in China since early times for the treatment of tuberculosis, malaria, and "female complaints."[2]

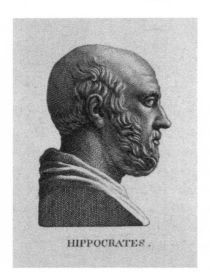

HIPPOCRATES .

Hippocrates, the "Father of Medicine," recommended arsenic compounds for the treatment of ulcers or sores on the body. *Courtesy of the National Library of Medicine.*

Although the discovery of white arsenic is often attributed to the Arab alchemist Jabir ibn Hayyan (eighth century AD), the compound was actually known to Greek alchemists by the early Christian era. It was readily obtained by roasting orpiment or realgar. White arsenic is quite toxic, and there does not appear to be any conclusive proof of its use in medicine before the eleventh century AD. At that time, the famous Persian physician ibn Sina, known to the West as Avicenna, recommended it (both internally and externally) for the treatment of cancer. Thereafter, salves containing arsenic were popular remedies for cancer. In general, the medieval Arabs made frequent use of arsenic ointments. Martin Levey's translation of a medical formulary by the ninth-century Arab physician and philosopher al-Kindī states that arsenic was used in the treatment of skin ulcers, decayed teeth, gum problems, and eye ailments.[3]

As R. P. Multhauf has pointed out, Arabs made significantly more use of minerals in therapeutics than ancient Greeks. This interest in the use of minerals, including arsenic, in medicine was transmitted to medieval European alchemists and medical chemists. As previously noted, however, it was Paracelsus and his followers who popularized the medicinal use of minerals such as arsenic and antimony beginning in the sixteenth century. Paracelsus believed that arsenic trioxide was effective in the treatment of cancers, wounds, and ulcers on the body, though he warned that this form of arsenic should only be used externally because of its toxicity. He also made medicinal use of a solution of potassium arsenate in alcohol that was similar to Fowler's solution. From the sixteenth through the eighteenth centuries, arsenic compounds were used to treat a variety of diseases, including plague, malaria, ulcers, and cancer. Arsenic may also have played an indirect role in medicine by helping to control the plague in this period through its use as a rat poison.[4]

John Haller has described how widespread the use of arsenic in therapeutics had become by the eighteenth century. He wrote:

> Throughout the eighteenth century, physicians prescribed arsenic both externally and internally. While pure metallic arsenic had no therapeutic use, its arsenides and salts were employed as alteratives [blood purifiers], antiseptics, antispasmodics, antiperiodics [prevent periodic return of diseases such as malaria], caustics [burn off tumors or other growths], cholagogues [promote bile flow], depilatories, hematinics [improve quality of blood], sedatives, and tonics. Some sixty different preparations were tried therapeutically in the history of its use, and probably twenty or more were still in circulation by the end of the nineteenth century, including Aiken's Tonic Pills, Andrew's Tonic, Arsenauro, Gross' Neuralgia Pills, Chloro-Phosphide of Arsenic, and Sulphur Compound Lozenges.

Numerous compounds of arsenic, such as copper arsenite, iron arsenate, sodium arsenate, and quinine arsenate, were used medicinally. Arsenic preparations were taken both externally and internally. As Haller has explained, the use of arsenic in therapeutics began to shift its emphasis from external to internal administration after the introduction of a procedure to make arsenic trioxide more soluble in water by boiling it with an alkali. This process led to the introduction of various solutions of arsenic compounds, the most popular and important of which was Fowler's solution.[5]

Fowler's Solution

Thomas Fowler was born in York, England, in 1736. From 1760 to 1764, he operated a pharmacy in York, and he then went to Edinburgh to earn his medical degree. He practiced medicine in Stafford, England, where he became physician for the General Infirmary of the county of Stafford.

In the early 1780s, a patent medicine known as Tasteless Ague and Fever Drops, whose formula was secret, was being used at the General Infirmary for the treatment of malaria (commonly called ague) and other intermittent fevers. The product claimed to be able to cure cases of malaria that even cinchona bark, the quinine-containing bark that was commonly used against malaria, was not effective against. It also did not have the bitter taste of cinchona and cost considerably less. Dr. Fowler suggested to the infirmary's apothecary, a man named Hughes, that he try to duplicate the formula of the patent medicine. Hughes found that arsenic was the active ingredient in the secret remedy, and he made up an arsenic solution that he hoped could take the place of the patent medicine. After testing the preparation on patients, Fowler made some modifications in its composition.[6]

In 1786 Fowler published an account of his preparation, *Medical Report of the Effects of Arsenic, in the Cure of Agues, Remitting Fevers, and Periodic Headaches.* Fowler's product essentially consisted of an aqueous solution of arsenic trioxide with a plant alkaloid (an alkaline or basic compound derived from a plant), with the alkaline substance making the arsenic trioxide more soluble in water. Later other alkaline substances, such as potassium carbonate or potassium nitrate, were generally used in place of alkaloids. Fowler called his concoction Solutio Mineralis (mineral solution), preferring not to specifically alert patients that the preparation contained arsenic. He was well aware that the public associated arsenic with poison and that it was best to avoid the term. In his 1786 book, Fowler reported remarkable results for his solution against ague. He concluded that: ". . . of two Hundred and forty-seven Cases, in which it was administered, two Hundred and forty-two have been radically cured, or had their Fits suspended, or relieved; I believe that very few Medicines, if any, are to be found among the Rank of Specifics, possessed of a more general curative Influence, than the *Mineral Solution* in *Agues*."[7]

After claiming that only five cases were not cured or relieved, he even hinted at a possible explanation for these failures: "It might be alleged that these five Patients only took the Solution from three to five Days each: this Argument however I shall not urge: infallible Remedies are not expected." When one examines Fowler's detailed discussion of the cases he treated, however, it is obvious, as James Whorton has pointed out, that the general conclusion cited above is somewhat misleading. For example, Fowler counted among his successes patients who did not respond to the solution but who later recovered upon being given cinchona bark, describing them as having been cured by "the Assistance of the Bark" (thus allowing some role for his solution in the cure). Also, his results were complicated by the periodic nature of the disease. Malaria attacks generally subside after a few weeks, although relapse is common. Although Fowler reported cases where relapses occurred, he still counted them in his 242 successful cases. In addition, Fowler did not count as failures patients who stopped coming to the clinic because they did not think they were improving. Patients also commonly suffered toxic side effects from the treatment, but Fowler did not believe these were serious enough to justify discontinuing the use of the medicine.[8]

Fowler's Solutio Mineralis eventually came to be called Fowler's solution. In 1809, it was included for the first time in the *London Pharmacopoeia*, the official drug compendium for England, under the name Liquor Arsenicalis. Beginning in 1819, it made its way into the pharmacopoeias of various European countries, and it was also included in the first edition of the *United States Pharmacopoeia* in 1822. The preparation found in most pharmacopoeias was a solution of arsenic trioxide in aqueous potassium carbonate, with "Fowler's solution" either as title or as a synonym. In other words, it was an aqueous solution of potassium arsenite.[9]

Fowler's solution quickly achieved widespread popularity in medicine. At the same time that the solution first appeared in the *London Pharmacopoeia*, British physician G. N. Hill wrote a series of articles praising arsenic and claiming that it had been neglected by physicians for too long because of concerns about its toxicity. Part of the difficulty with the use of arsenic in the past, according to Hill, was that doctors had used doses of the medicine that were too large, and he advocated its responsible use in doses small enough to cure but not to injure. He argued that the medical community should be grateful to Fowler for providing this remedy, which was both a tonic and a stimulant. Hill recommended the use of the medication, alone or in combination with other drugs, for a host of diseases and conditions, including malaria, epilepsy, hysteria, morbid changes in the liver and spleen, rheumatism, heart palpitations, and syphilis.

Not all physicians, however, heeded Hill's admonition to give the remedy in small doses. The early nineteenth century was a period when many physicians believed in a "heroic therapy" involving the use of aggressive bloodletting and large doses of powerful drugs such as the cathartic (laxative) calomel (mercurous chloride). One American physician, for example, argued that arsenic must often be given in increasing doses to the points where signs of toxicity are manifested. British physicians Thomas Hunt and James Begbie were two other ardent supporters of Fowler's solution who, while admitting that some physicians had been careless in its use, argued for its great value as a therapeutic agent. Both urged that the drug be used discreetly but claimed that in most cases it would need to be administered for days or even weeks, often resulting in some toxic side effects.[10]

Fowler's solution was used for so many purposes that it was referred to by one American physician as one of medicine's "therapeutic mules." In addition to the diseases mentioned above, it was also used for the treatment of asthma, chorea (a condition of involuntary spasmodic movements of facial muscles or limbs), diphtheria, lymphoma, worms, typhus, and many other illnesses. One textbook of the late nineteenth century identified arsenic as the most extensively used internal medicine for dermatological problems. In fact, it remained a treatment for psoriasis until the middle of the twentieth century. Because of the belief in its tonic (or stimulant) properties, one physician even expressed the opinion that it should be given several days before any major operation to increase survival rates.[11]

Fowler's solution continued to hold a place in medicine well into the twentieth century. By 1940 or so, however, its use began to decline, and the last edition of the *United States Pharmacopeia* in which it appeared was in 1950 (although other arsenic compounds continued to be included). Fowler's solution was still being used to some extent in dermatology and certain other areas at least until the 1960s. Prolonged or excessive use of the drug could result in cancer or other problems. At least as late as the 1980s, for example, there were reports in the medical literature of patients diagnosed with hepatic or lung cancer induced by Fowler's solution.[12]

Although Fowler's solution was by far the most popular form in which arsenic was administered during the nineteenth century, it was by no means the only arsenic-containing medication. James Whorton has summarized the extensive use of arsenic in Victorian medicine as follows:

> Practitioners also had recourse to Pearson's solution (potassium arsenate), Donovan's solution (arsenic iodide), Bieto's solution (ammonium arsenate), de Valagin's solution (arsenious acid dissolved in hydrochloric acid), and still other solutions. In the 1840s, arsenic was discovered to be present in the springs of spas such as Bath, where people had long treated multiple ailments by taking the waters. . . . Nor were arsenic preparations limited to liquids. The oldest dosage form of all—the external application of arsenicals as pastes or salves, favoured by the physicians of antiquity—also continued in use, as a depilatory and to remove warts and moles. Arsenic was given as pills, inhaled as vapour, taken by enema, and, after the hypodermic syringe was introduced in the 1850s, received by injection.[13]

The use of arsenic in medicine was no doubt given a boost by reports of the arsenic eaters of Styria about the middle of the nineteenth century.

Arsenic Eaters of Styria

In 1851 the medical world learned of the practice of arsenic eating among peasants in Styria (now a region of Austria) through the publication of an article in a Viennese medical journal. The author was a Swiss physician, naturalist, and traveler named Johann Jakob von Tschudi, who had spent five years traveling in the Andes beginning in 1838. Tschudi published books on his travels in Peru and on the fauna of that country in the 1840s. He later spent several years traveling in various parts of South America, and he served as Switzerland's ambassador to Brazil from 1860 to 1868.[14]

According to Tschudi, the stimulus for his 1851 paper was a trial involving a poisoning case that had recently taken place in the town of Cilli, part of Austria-Hungary. During the trial, the question was raised as to whether or not a certain military officer was a "toxicophagus." Tschudi went on to say that since the "toxicophagi" were "more or less unknown to the medical public, I have thought it my duty to publish some information and observations on the subject." He does not specify exactly how this issue was raised in the trial, but it seems likely from what follows that the officer was a victim of arsenic poisoning and that a question arose as to whether the accused poisoned him or whether he had taken the arsenic himself.[15]

Tschudi explained that the so-called toxicophagi were a group of peasants in Styria and Lower Austria who were in the habit of eating arsenic. They purchased the arsenic under various names (e.g., hedri or hedrich) from itinerant herbalists and peddlers. Their purpose in taking the arsenic was either to acquire a fresh complexion and appearance of flourishing health or to facilitate respiration when walking or working in the mountainous terrain of the area. Tschudi noted that these toxicophagi began by taking a small piece of the arsenic about the size of a lentil (less than half a grain) several times a week. After a period of time, they gradually increased the dose as the smaller quantity lost its effect. Tschudi gives an example of a roughly sixty-year-old man who had increased the dose over time to about four grains (enough to kill most people).

Tschudi also reported that the toxicophagi became dependent on the arsenic and suffered ill consequences if they ceased using it. The symptoms of withdrawal that he described included anxiety, indigestion, loss of appetite, vomiting, constipation, and spasmodic pain. Although arsenic eaters appeared to develop a certain tolerance for the poison, and many showed no signs of chronic poisoning, Tschudi pointed out that the number of deaths from abuse of arsenic was not trifling.

It was not clear how many of the peasants were arsenic eaters nor how many deaths could be attributed to this practice. The law forbade the illegal possession of arsenic, and so many of the toxicophagi concealed their habit. Tschudi also noted that grooms and coachmen, even in the city of Vienna, commonly gave arsenic to horses in order to give them a glossy, round, and elegant appearance, and also to increase their respiratory capacity.

Tschudi's original German article was translated into English and French in several medical journals. It was also brought to the attention of the broader English-speaking public through an article in *Chambers's Journal of Popular Literature, Science and Arts* in 1856 and through a discussion of the subject in James Johnston's popular 1855 book, *The Chemistry of Popular Life*. Johnston's romantic description of the arsenic eaters was already mentioned in the discussion of arsenic as a cosmetic in the preceding chapter. Tschudi himself, stimulated by the interest his article had generated and the doubts expressed about the arsenic eaters in several English medical journals, published a further paper on the subject in 1853, expanding upon his earlier observations.[16]

But medical writers, especially in Britain, continued by and large to be skeptical of Tschudi's account of the toxicophagi. Physician W. B. Kesteven, for example, wrote a three-part article in the journal of the British Medical Association in 1856 in which he translated Tschudi's article and then proceeded to attack it and the accounts based on it. He argued that much of the evidence for arsenic eating was based on hearsay rather than on any systematic observation of the so-called arsenic eaters over an extended period of time. He criticized those who wrote these accounts as either not being medically trained (such as the chemist Johnston) or not having substantial clinical experience (such as Tschudi, whom he characterized as more of a traveler than a doctor). Kesteven also pointed out that no chemical analysis of the substance ingested by the Styrian peasants had been made in order to confirm that it was arsenic. Finally, he cited the opinions of noted British toxicologists such as Jonathan Pereira, Robert Christison, and Alfred Taylor, all of whom dismissed the story of the arsenic eaters as a fable.[17]

The debate over the arsenic eaters continued, however, and several individuals attempted to obtain further evidence of the practice. In 1860 Charles Heisch, a lecturer in chemistry at Middlesex Hospital in England, addressed questions about the practice to several physicians living in Styria with whom he was acquainted. He collected their first-hand accounts of arsenic eaters in the region and published the results of his inquiries in an article in the *Pharmaceutical Journal*. In that same year, Henry Enfield Roscoe, professor of chemistry at Owens University in Manchester, delivered a paper on arsenic eating before the Manchester Literary and Philosophical Society that was eventually published in 1862. Roscoe communicated with seventeen physicians in Styria who sent him information on cases of arsenic eating that they had personally observed or that had been related to them by "trustworthy persons." In addition, Roscoe obtained from one of his correspondents a sample of a substance that had been taken from a farm laborer who was caught secretly eating it. Roscoe analyzed the sample and determined that it was white arsenic. He ended his paper by concluding, "That arsenious acid [white arsenic] is taken regularly into the system, by certain persons in Styria, in quantities usually supposed sufficient to produce immediate death."[18]

The strongest evidence that Roscoe presented, however, was taken from a paper sent to him by the author, Dr. Schäfer of Graz, which described a case under the personal examination of another physician, Dr. Knappe. In the presence of the doctor, a thirty-year-old woodcutter in good health who had been consuming arsenic for twelve years ate a piece of white arsenic weighing 4.5 grains (considered to be a lethal dose). On the following day, he consumed another 5.5 grains of the poison. He informed the doctor that he was in the habit of taking this amount of arsenic three or four times a week. The doctor examined his urine on two occasions and found arsenic present in both cases. The man ate with his normal appetite, drank liquor freely, and appeared to be in good health.[19]

Further evidence of arsenic eating was provided by Scottish physician Craig Maclagan, who traveled to Styria with a colleague to investigate the subject and published his results in the *Edinburgh Medical Journal* in 1864. While in Styria, he visited Knappe, who arranged for him to meet with two arsenic eaters in the village of Liegist.

The first arsenic eater was a twenty-six-year-old man who appeared to be in good health and who worked as a house servant. The young man informed the doctor that he took orpiment, or yellow arsenic, twice a week and that he experienced a longing for the chemical if he went without it for two weeks. He generally used yellow arsenic because it was easier to obtain than white arsenic. In the presence of Maclagan and Knappe, the man consumed a quantity of powdered white arsenic weighing between four and five grains spread on a piece of bread. Maclagan collected and analyzed samples of his urine, which did contain arsenic. The man showed no ill effects from the arsenic on the following day.

The second case involved a forty-six-year-old-tailor, also in good health, who had been taking arsenic (usually in the form of orpiment) for fifteen years. In the presence of the doctors, he consumed about six grains of pow-dered white arsenic on a piece of bread. The tailor informed the physicians that he was in the habit of taking this amount of arsenic, or more, every four to eight days. He indicated that he felt a craving for another dose if he did not take it for two weeks. The man showed no ill effects from his habit, and once again his urine tested positive for arsenic.

Although Maclagan admitted that some of the physiological actions attributed to arsenic by those who consumed it were probably "fanciful," he believed that he had demonstrated the existence of people who regularly consumed the poison in doses considered to be lethal. He also concluded that he has established humans' ability to build up a tolerance to arsenic.[20]

A decade later, Knappe provided additional proof of the existence of arsenic eaters at a German scientific meeting in 1875. After delivering some remarks on the subject, he introduced two Styrian peasants. In the presence of those attending the meeting, one of the men consumed four to six grains of yellow arsenic, and the other six grains of white arsenic. On the following day, Knappe again exhibited the two men to his colleagues, showing they were still healthy.[21]

Although there were some who remained skeptical, the medical and scientific literature of the late nineteenth and early twentieth centuries suggests that many physicians and chemists came to accept the validity of the accounts of the Styrian arsenic eaters. For example, in the 1905 edition of his textbook of chemistry, Henry Roscoe repeated his belief that arsenic eating was a fact, arguing that there were well-authenticated cases of the practice. An article in the *British Medical Journal* in 1901 claimed, "It is a matter of common knowledge that arsenic and its salts exhibited for a time in small doses establish a tolerance, and the arsenic eaters of the Austrian Tyrol are the classical proofs of the fact."[22]

Efforts to prove or disprove the ability to develop a tolerance to arsenic continued in the twentieth century. For example, Swiss pharmacologist Max Cloetta claimed to have produced tolerance to arsenic in dogs and rabbits in 1906, although further studies five years later convinced him that this tolerance was more apparent than real. Erich Schwartze, head of the Pharmacological Laboratory of the Bureau of Chemistry carried out extensive laboratory animal research in the 1920s and concluded that he had demonstrated "the improbability of developing any noteworthy systemic or gastrointestinal habituation to 'arsenic' by feeding—the only manner in which habituation to 'arsenic' has been claimed to have been produced in man or laboratory mammals." In that same decade, Harvard entomologist F. L.

Campbell showed that tolerance to arsenic "was not induced in silkworms by quantitative feeding of sublethal doses of sodium arsenate solutions."[23]

More recent studies have provided stronger evidence for the development of tolerance to arsenic in certain animals and even in human cells. Some plants have also been shown to be unusually tolerant to arsenic.[24] In his recent book on arsenic, chemist William Cullen concluded, "Because the number of arsenic eaters in Styria was relatively small, and because they were very secretive about their habit, it was difficult to unequivocally prove their existence. Nevertheless, there is a considerable body of scientific evidence that Styrian peasants did deliberately ingest poisonous arsenic trioxide."[25]

Some writers believe that arsenic eating by humans actually evolved out of the feeding of the chemical to horses to increase their strength and improve their health, a practice possibly initiated by gypsies. The custom of feeding of arsenic to horses was not confined to Austria but spread over time to other countries. Cullen has observed: "Prominent Australian veterinarian Percy Sykes recently said that arsenic was widely used as a tonic in the 1930s and 90 per cent of horses would have had it in their systems."[26]

In fact, one theory of the 1932 death of the most famous horse in Australian racing history, Phar Lap, involves arsenic poisoning. It has been suggested that Phar Lap was poisoned on orders from American gangsters concerned that he would affect their gambling revenues. The horse was so famous that his body was stuffed and displayed in the Melbourne Museum in Australia. In 2006 samples of the horse's hair were analyzed using X-ray spectroscopy, and arsenic was found in the "skin end" of the samples. Investigators noted that these findings were consistent with a large dose of arsenic given a day or two before the horse's death. Several explanations besides murder, however, might explain the presence of the arsenic. For example, it is possible that Phar Lap ate vegetation treated with an arsenic pesticide, that he was given an accidental overdose of an arsenical tonic, or that arsenic was used by the taxidermist to help preserve the body.[27]

Sleeping Sickness, Syphilis, and Salvarsan

As previously indicated, arsenic compounds had been tried in the treatment of various infectious diseases, such as malaria and plague. The first scientific demonstration of the effectiveness of arsenic against certain microorganisms, however, concerned the microbes known as trypanosomes in the late nineteenth and early twentieth centuries. Trypanosomes are a type of protozoa that cause sleeping sickness and other diseases. Sleeping sickness was a major public health problem in Africa in the nineteenth century and has undergone a resurgence on that continent in recent decades after being nearly eradicated in the 1960s. The Scottish missionary and explorer David Livingstone was the first person to suggest, in 1852, that the cattle disease nagana (an animal infection similar to human sleeping sickness) was transmitted by the bite of the tsetse fly. It was not until 1895, however, that another Scottish investigator, pathologist and microbiologist David Bruce, discovered that a trypanosome was the cause of nagana. In 1901 British colonial physician Robert Michael Forde discovered an organism in the blood of an infected steamboat captain, but he erroneously identified it as a worm. A few months later, English physician Joseph Everett Dutton correctly identified the organism as a trypanosome, providing the first strong evidence that sleeping sickness in humans was also caused by this organism. About the same time, Italian physician Aldo Castellani identified trypanosomes in the cerebrospinal fluid of sleeping sickness patients. Shortly thereafter, it was shown conclusively that the trypanosome causing the disease was transmitted by tsetse flies.[28]

The first attempt to use arsenic for the treatment of trypanosomiasis (a trypanosome infection) appears to have been made by the aforementioned David Livingstone. He claimed that he had used arsenic to treat an animal with nagana in 1847 or 1848, but the results were not definitive, and he did not publish them. In 1858, stimulated by Livingstone's account of nagana and the tsetse fly in his *Missionary Travels and Researches in South Africa*, James Braid suggested in a letter to the *British Medical Journal* that Livingstone should try arsenic against this disease. Braid's belief in the possible efficacy of this treatment was based on reports in the literature that arsenic could protect against the bite of a poisonous snake. At this time, the role of the trypanosome in causing the disease was not known, and perhaps Braid thought that the tsetse fly injected venom into the animal that it bit.[29]

The next advance came when French physician Charles Louis Laveran reported in 1902 that he had found sodium arsenite to be effective in treating

158 KING OF POISONS

trypanosomes in infected laboratory animals. Unfortunately, the effect of the chemical was short lived, and the organism reappeared in the blood of the animals within a few days, ultimately leading to their deaths. Hopes were raised again three years later when H. Wolferstan Thomas, an investigator at the Liverpool School of Tropical Medicine, published the encouraging results of his research on the use of an organic arsenic compound named atoxyl in nagana. He described how he came to try this drug in an effort to find a relatively nontoxic arsenic drug for treating trypanosomiasis: "An aniline compound, meta-arsenaureanilid (atoxyl), having the formula $C_6H_6NO_2As$, attracted my attention. This preparation had been before the profession since 1900, and various workers have recorded its worth in the treatment of various skin affections and in anemia. . . . It produces no necrosis, no pain, and very much higher doses of arsenic can be given without producing toxic results. (I have tried the drug in high doses intravenously on myself without ill effects.)"[30]

Thomas was fortunate that he did not suffer any ill effects from the atoxyl, for it was soon shown that the drug was far from benign. When trying the drug against sleeping sickness in East Africa, for example, Robert Koch stated that about 2 percent of the patients went blind through atrophy of the optic nerve. Relapses also commonly occurred. Atoxyl was thus not the hoped-for cure for trypanosomiasis.[31]

The first successful arsenic compound for the treatment of trypanosomiais was developed by the German physician and scientist Paul Ehrlich. Ehrlich was born into a German-Jewish family in 1854. He obtained his medical degree from the University of Leipzig in 1878 for a thesis on the staining of animal tissues with dyes, a subject that held his interest for many years. In 1890 he joined the staff of Robert Koch's Institute for Infectious Diseases in Berlin, where he did important work in immunology. In fact, he received a Nobel Prize in Medicine or Physiology in 1908 for his immunological research. But Ehrlich was also interested in the possibility of using synthetic chemical drugs to attack pathogenic (disease-causing) microorganisms in the human host. His interest in dyes led him to first try dyestuffs such as trypan red against the trypanosomes that caused sleeping sickness and other diseases. The studies of Laveran and others on arsenic drugs stimulated Ehrlich to also investigate the therapeutic potential of these compounds. In fact, he actually tested atoxyl in 1903 but rejected it because it did not kill try-panosomes in the test tube. The demonstration by Thomas that atoxyl could eliminate trypanosomes from the bloodstream led Ehrlich to take another look at the compound.

Although atoxyl had been shown to be too toxic for use in humans and higher animals, Ehrlich reasoned that it should be possible to decrease its

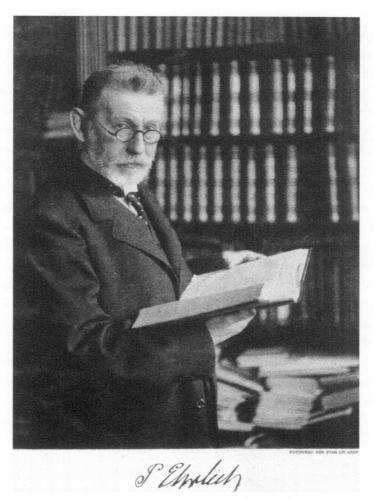

**Paul Ehrlich developed the organic arsenic drug Salvarsan, which
became the standard treatment for syphilis until the introduction of penicillin.**
Courtesy of the National Library of Medicine.

toxicity to the host animal by modification of the chemical structure of the molecule without decreasing its toxicity toward trypanosomes. Ehrlich was one of the pioneers in the field of drug design based on systematically modifying the structure of a molecule in order to alter its pharmacological action. He was the founder of modern chemotherapy, which he defined as the search for synthetic chemicals to treat infectious diseases. Others later broadened the term to include the use of chemicals against essentially any type of disease (e.g., cancer). By the time that he began his intensive study of arsenic compounds, he was the head of his own research institute, where he and his colleagues tested hundreds of chemicals that they had synthesized or obtained from the pharmaceutical and chemical industry.

Ehrlich's search for a successful therapeutic agent was not based simply on random testing of chemical compounds. He observed the properties of various compounds, especially their toxicity against and affinity for human cells and trypanosomes, and then instructed his staff to make specific changes in the chemical structures of the molecules in order to achieve his desired goal of a drug that would kill trypanosomes within the human body without doing serious harm to the host. Although a kind and compassionate man, he carefully directed and controlled all of the work in the laboratory, sometimes causing resentment among senior colleagues who believed they should have more independence. Every morning, Ehrlich would provide staff members with specific instructions for their day's work. He once complained to a colleague of the difficulty of finding skilled and independent scientists who at the same time would be inclined to acquiesce in his ideas and develop them therapeutically.

Ehrlich's instructions to his coworkers were written on cards of different colors that he called "blocks," and he kept copies of them in a "duplicate book." One problem for his coworkers, who knew that Ehrlich expected them to follow these instructions implicitly, was that his handwriting was almost illegible. Fortunately, one staff member had become somewhat of an expert in reading Ehrlich's handwriting, and his coworkers frequently brought him their "blocks" to decipher.

Given Ehrlich's careful control of the experiments in his laboratory, one might have expected that he maintained a neat and well-organized office, but nothing could be further from the truth. His secretary of many years,

Martha Marquardt, gave the following description of Ehrlich's private laboratory and office:

> It was evident that no one ever sat on the sofa, except perhaps in the very earliest days of the Institute. Later on it was obviously destined to bear only the heavy burden of the high piles of books placed upon it. The whole seat was covered with heaps of books, periodicals, documents and writings, some in large envelopes, others in large blue cardboard folders. The top of the writing-desk, the little table in the opposite corner and the bookstand beneath the window had suffered the same fate, as had the two chairs in front of the bookshelves, and also these themselves.

In spite of this disarray, however, Marquardt claimed that Ehrlich could always find any important document or manuscript from the piles on the sofa and other furniture.[32]

The first organic arsenic compound tested in Ehrlich's laboratory that yielded any significant results against trypanosomes was compound number 418 (the 418th compound to be tested). The search continued, however, for a better therapeutic agent. After the microorganism that caused syphilis was identified in 1905, several investigators began to try arsenic compounds against syphilis in the mistaken belief that the spirochetes that cause this disease were very similar to trypanosomes. Although Ehrlich did not at first carry out experiments on syphilis, he did arrange for a colleague to test arsenicals that showed the most promise against trypanosomes on syphilis in monkeys and apes.

In 1909 Sahachiro Hata, who had carried out syphilis experiments with rabbits in Japan, came to work in Ehrlich's laboratory. Ehrlich set him to work testing the effects of numerous compounds on syphilis and relapsing fever (a disease caused by a trypanosome). When Hata tested compound number 606 on experimental animals, he found it to be an effective antisyphilitic agent. The compound had actually been synthesized in 1907, but the assistant who tested it at the time against trypanosomes did not report any significant therapeutic results. It is not clear why he obtained these negative results, for the compound was soon shown to be useful in the treatment of trypanosomal diseases as well as syphilis.

After extensive animal tests, limited supplies of 606 were distributed to selected specialists for clinical trials. The results were encouraging enough for Ehrlich to announce the discovery of 606 at a medical congress in 1910. The announcement was greeted with great enthusiasm, particularly with respect to its effectiveness against syphilis. The demand for the drug soon outgrew the ability of Ehrlich's laboratory to produce it. Ehrlich then arranged with a German chemical firm to manufacture 606, which was patented under the trade name Salvarsan. It was by no means an ideal drug. As an arsenic compound, Salvarsan had some significant side effects, and the treatment of syphilis with the drug usually involved weekly injections for a year or more. Nevertheless, it represented the first practical success for Ehrlich's concept of chemotherapy and was a milestone in the treatment of syphilis.[33]

Although a great deal of praise was heaped on Ehrlich for the discovery of Salvarsan, he and the drug were also subject to criticism. In addition to legitimate questions raised by medical authorities about the evidence supporting the effectiveness of Salvarsan or its potential side effects, opponents attacked Ehrlich on the basis of opposition to the use of chemical remedies and of anti-Semitism. They made greatly exaggerated claims about the number of fatalities and cases of serious injury such as blindness that could be attributed to the use of the drug. Ehrlich, a sensitive man, was hurt by these charges and did his best to refute them.

One particularly unpleasant incident actually led to a court case in which Ehrlich was reluctantly forced to testify as an expert witness. In 1913 a man named Karl Wassmann, a strange character who privately published a newspaper called *The Free-Thinker* that he often distributed in cafes while dressed in a monk's cowl and sandals, began a series of attacks on Salvarsan, condemning Ehrlich and the physicians who used the drug. As Baümler explained:

> This stance was prompted initially by a purely local affair. Prostitutes and pimps had complained to Wassmann that an untested drug, Salvarsan, was being given to prostitutes against their will in the Frankfurt Hospital. This suggested to Wassmann that the Director of the Dermatology Department [where syphilis was treated], Professor Hexheimer, and his senior physician were nothing more than profit-seeking entrepreneurs, whose greed even led to premeditated murder.

He also suggested that the Salvarsan business was simply a cover for financial machinations.[34]

Wassmann also claimed that most of the patients receiving the drug suffered from severe side effects, such as blindness and paralysis, and that some even died as a result of the treatment. Ehrlich and the pharmaceutical company that manufactured Salvarsan decided not to take any action against Wassmann for the attacks. The director of the Frankfurt Hospital, however, brought charges against Wassmann, leading to a trial. The government also brought charges against Wassmann in the public interest. These proceedings greatly distressed Ehrlich.

In the end, the court concluded that the charges made by Wassmann were false, and he was found guilty and sentenced to a year in prison. At the trial, he was revealed to have accepted money from some of the prostitutes involved for writing the articles, a fact that no doubt also counted against him. Wassmann actually served only two months of his sentence because he was released under the amnesty declared at the outbreak of World War I.

Although Salvarsan was praised for its effectiveness in the treatment of syphilis, efforts continued to develop a better and safer arsenical drug to treat the disease. Ehrlich himself developed a somewhat improved version of the drug, which he called Neosalvarsan, before his death in 1915. In the 1930s another organic arsenic compound, Mapharsen, which could be given in smaller doses than Salvarsan or Neosalvarsan and had fewer side effects than these substances, was added to the arsenal of anti-syphilitic drugs.[35]

Another development of the 1930s was the introduction of rapid treatment methods for syphilis. One of the problems involved in the treatment of the disease with Salvarsan and other arsenicals was the issue of patient compliance. A course of weekly injections for a year or more was too much of a burden for many patients, and often they did not complete the full course of treatment. Clinicians at Mount Sinai Hospital in New York developed a procedure for administering arsenicals continuously by slow intravenous drip, although the patients had to be hospitalized. Other so-called rapid treatment methods, such as repeated injections of arsenicals over a period of a few days or weeks, were introduced as well, but these also required close medical supervision. These new procedures greatly reduced the length of the treatment.[36]

When the United States entered World War II, the government established a series of rapid treatment centers near military training camps and
important war industry facilities. Their purpose was to serve as quarantine
hospitals for prostitutes and "promiscuous" women with venereal diseases,
whom the government saw as a threat to the war effort because they could
infect servicemen and essential war industry workers. Skeptical that these
women would complete the lengthy outpatient treatment for syphilis, the
government decided to quarantine the women and subject them to rapid
treatment methods to cure their disease and render them noninfectious.[37]

With the introduction of penicillin as a therapeutic agent and the demonstration of its effectiveness against syphilis during the Second World War,
the use of arsenical drugs to treat the disease was abandoned. Penicillin
quickly, effectively, and safely treated syphilis. Arsenical drugs still continued
to be used, however, for other purposes in medicine.[38]

Arsenic in Dentistry

The use of arsenic in treating dental problems goes back to ancient times.
Chinese medical works from before the common era, for example, recommended packing arsenic sulfide paste around diseased teeth in order to
encourage necrosis of the tissue so that the tooth would fall out. Ancient
Chinese practitioners also reportedly placed pellets of arsenic in painful
teeth to kill a "tooth worm." Arabs in the Middle Ages also used arsenic compounds to promote tooth loss, as well as to coat the roots of teeth to be
extracted and to ease the pain of toothache.

As dentistry emerged as a modern profession in the nineteenth century,
arsenic remained one of the medications used in dental practice. Dr. John
Roach Spooner of Montreal, Canada, is generally credited with the use of
arsenic trioxide to kill the pulp (the soft material inside the tooth that contains
nerves and blood vessels) of infected teeth, although his discovery was not
recorded until his brother Shearjashub, a New York dentist, published it in
1836 in his *Guide to Sound Teeth*. In this way, the pain could be relieved without
pulling the tooth. On the use of arsenic for this purpose, Shearjashub Spooner
wrote, "So complete and satisfactory is the operation of arsenic in destroying
the living fibre, that, instead of extracting teeth whenever the nerve is badly

exposed, we destroy it, plug the teeth, and thus preserve them. Teeth thus treated will often last a great number of years, and prove highly serviceable."[39]

Although some critics warned that this practice was dangerous, by 1850, according to Whorton, "it was standard practice among dentists to apply to painful pulp a mixture of creosote, morphine, and arsenic."[40] The procedure worked well for some patients, but not for others. One danger was that the arsenic could kill more than the pulp and damage the tooth socket or the gums. John Hyson has explained that the safety of using arsenic improved after the introduction of gutta-percha, an elastic natural latex produced by the tree of the same name, in the 1840s. This substance was used to seal the cavity and help prevent the arsenic from leaking out and causing damage to surrounding tissues. Gutta-percha is still sometimes used in dentistry today for filling the empty space inside the root of a tooth after it has undergone a root canal procedure.

The use of arsenic in dentistry remained controversial. The topic was the subject of a heated debate, for example, at the ninth annual meeting of the American Society of Dental Surgeons in Saratoga, New York, in 1848. In the 1890s, whether dentists should use arsenic became largely a moot point as cocaine hydrochloride anesthesia began to replace arsenic as the drug of choice for the eradication of pulp. Yet arsenic did not completely disappear from dentistry in the twentieth century. Although the majority of the profession would agree that there is no longer any indication for the use of arsenic in dental practice today, there are occasional reports in the recent literature of injuries due to the use of arsenic by dentists.[41]

Arsenic in the Treatment of Cancer

It is ironic that arsenic, which is a well-documented carcinogen (although some authorities apparently still do not concede this fact), should also turn out to be useful in the treatment of cancer. We have already seen that arsenic was tried as a remedy against certain cancers at least since medieval times, and perhaps earlier. Various arsenic pastes and ointments were commonly used for the external treatment of cancers in the eighteenth and nineteenth centuries, and Fowler's solution was also used against the disease after its introduction. It is not clear that these treatments were efficacious.

Arsenic's major success came in the treatment of leukemia. The first documented report of the use of arsenic in leukemia was published by a German physician named Lissauer in 1865. He administered the drug to a woman with chronic myeloid leukemia (CML), and she was restored to health, but only temporarily. In 1878 American physicians E. G. Cutler and E. H. Bradford reported on their study of the effects of arsenic on blood cells. They found that Fowler's solution produced a decline in the white blood cell count, although it also reduced the red blood cell count. In a patient with CML treated with arsenic for ten weeks, the reduction in the white blood cell count was dramatic. As Lissauer found, however, the white blood cell count increased, and hence the patient relapsed, when the arsenic therapy was discontinued. Arsenic therapy became the main treatment for leukemia until it was replaced by radiation therapy in the early twentieth century.[42]

Arsenic did make a short-lived comeback for the treatment of CML in the 1930s, however. As Waxman and Anderson explained:

It then experienced a brief resurgence in popularity following a report in 1931 of nine patients with CML who responded to arsenic trioxide therapy at Boston City Hospital. Laboratory and clinical changes included reduction in total white blood cell counts from several hundred thousand per milliliter to an approximately normal, reduction in the size of enlarged livers and spleens, a return to apparently normal hematopoiesis [formation of blood cells] in bone marrow biopsy specimens, and a sense of well being. Discontinuation of therapy was followed by clinical and hematologic relapse within weeks.

Within a few years, however, it was discovered that arsenic trioxide therapy could result in chronic arsenic poisoning and required careful patient monitoring. The use of this drug then declined, to be replaced by radiotherapy and cytotoxic (cell-killing) chemotherapy.[43]

The use of arsenic to treat leukemia, however, was still not dead. Arsenic has a long history of use in traditional Chinese medicine, and the renewed use of arsenic to treat leukemia arose from the work of a folk healer in rural China. During the Cultural Revolution of the 1970s, Chairman Mao Tse-tung sent Western-trained doctors from the cities to rural areas of China to learn about traditional Chinese medicine. One of these doctors, Zhang Tingdong, arrived with a team of physicians in a remote agricultural commune in 1972. There they met an old medicine man working out of a primitive mud home. Zhang later described what they observed about one of the remedies employed by the folk healer: "What the doctor did have, though, was a powdery home-brewed concoction he'd learned from his father, made from two types of ground rock and the venom of a local toad. Some patients drank it; others rubbed it on their skin. To the visitors' surprise, it soon became clear that some of the patients—even some with cancer—got better, and some even seemed cured."[44]

Zhang took the ingredients and the recipe of the medicine back to Harbin Medical University, where he was based. He found that the toad venom was biologically very complex, that one rock consisted largely of mercury, and that the other rock contained high levels of arsenic trioxide. After animal testing and clinical trials on patients with leukemia, Zhang determined that it was the arsenic that was the active ingredient. Testing on many patients was required, however, before doctors could establish the appropriate dose of the medicine. Although Zhang published a paper on the subject, his work was largely ignored at the time. It was not until he collaborated with investigators at a prominent institute in Shanghai in the 1990s that the value of the drug became widely recognized. As Rosenthal explained, "The Shanghai specialists, scientists with research funding and international reputations, tried arsenic trioxide from Harbin with these [leukemia] patients, and they were awed. They began more technical studies on the drug than were possible in Harbin. And they spread the word abroad."[45]

The specific type of leukemia against which arsenic trioxide was especially efficacious was known as acute promyelocytic leukemia (APL). It is a relatively rare but especially unpleasant form of the disease involving anemia and susceptibility to infection and hemorrhages. In the 1990s, the introduction of trans-retinoic acid greatly improved the prognosis for APL patients. Studies in the 1990s in China and elsewhere demonstrated not only that arsenic trioxide was extremely effective in treating APL but also that it could produce remissions in patients who had relapsed after trans-retinoic acid treatment, a group that previously had not fared well unless given bone marrow transplantations. In the United States, arsenic trioxide was approved by the FDA in 2000. Arsenic is now used not only as a second line of defense in APL after trans-retinoic acid therapy but also in combination with the latter drug or by itself as a first-line therapy. In addition, the results of some recent studies have suggested that arsenic may be useful in treating other forms of cancer, such as multiple myeloma. There were some twenty-five ongoing clinical trials at the National Institutes of Health in 2007 involving the use of arsenic compounds against a variety of cancers.[46]

Arsenic and Homeopathy

In the late eighteenth century, a German physician named Samuel Hahnemann created an alternative system of medicine called homeopathy. Hahnemann's system was based on two main principles. The first was the so-called law of similars, which claimed that one should treat the symptoms of a disease by giving in small doses substances that in larger amount would cause those same symptoms. Thus, if one symptom of a disease was vomiting, then the physician should give the patient a small dose of a substance that would ordinarily induce vomiting. The second principle stated, against scientific reasoning and common sense, that the smaller the dose of the drug, the more potent its therapeutic effect would be. Hahnemann devised an elaborate system of diluting medicines to increase their strength, or "potentiate" them. Eventually, he recommended the use of drugs of the thirtieth dilution (each dilution being one to one hundred). As the noted pharmacologist A. J. Clark later wrote, "This works out at a content of 1 molecule of drug in a sphere with a circumference equal to the orbit of Neptune."[47]

Homeopaths argued that during the dilution process, the energy and efficacy of the drug molecule was transferred to the dilution medium. Homeopathy was relatively popular in nineteenth-century Europe and America, and although it became largely moribund in the early twentieth century thanks in large part to advances in medical science, it has undergone a resurgence in recent times. Homeopathy today exists in various forms, not all of which adhere strictly to Hahnemann's precepts.[48]

It is ironic, considering that homeopaths of the nineteenth century attacked orthodox physicians for their therapeutic use of strong minerals with serious toxic side effects (such as mercury compounds), that arsenic should have become one of the mainstays of homeopathic therapy. Of course, homeopathy called for its use in extremely minute doses. Arsenic trioxide, or Arsenicum album, as it was generally called by homeopaths, was prescribed for a wide variety of ailments. In his 1880 work on homeopathic materia medica, the prominent American homeopathic physician Constantine Hering claimed that arsenic was one of the first "provings" (i.e., a homeopathic method of testing a substance), although Hahnemann had not mentioned this drug in the first volume of his own treatise on materia medica (1811). In the second volume of Hahnemann's materia medica, published in 1816, he stated that he had not included arsenic in the earlier volume because he was concerned that frightened people would label him a "poison doctor." By 1839, in the second edition of his book on chronic diseases, Hahnemann listed 1,231 symptoms produced by arsenic, the basis for determining its therapeutic uses. Hering himself devoted some 66 pages to listing all of the effects of Arsenicum album, touching on virtually every system of the body.[49]

Arsenicum album as a homeopathic remedy is readily available in stores and on the Internet today. A recent textbook of homeopathic pharmacy lists more than a dozen indications for Arsenicum. Many of these relate to emotional or mental problems, such as being fearful (of being alone, the dark, etc.), restless, highly strung, insecure, or overly sensitive. Other conditions for which Arsenicum is recommended include headaches with nausea and vomiting, stinging eyes or nasal discharge, bleeding gums, mouth ulcers, and fevers involving sepsis (blood infection).[50]

Although in theory the amount of arsenic in homeopathic preparations should be small enough to do no harm, this does not appear to always be the case. Occasional reports of arsenic toxicity from taking arsenical homeopathic preparations have appeared in the literature. It may be in these cases that the remedy was incorrectly prepared or improperly used.[51]

Although it makes perfect sense with respect to homeopathic theory, it contradicts orthodox Western medicine to suggest that arsenic be used to treat people suffering from arsenic poisoning, yet that is exactly what some Indian scientists have recommended. As discussed in the previous chapter, millions of people in Bangladesh and parts of India are being exposed daily to drinking water containing high amounts of arsenic, and many are showing signs of chronic arsenic poisoning. Researchers from the Department of

Zoology at the University of Kalyani in India have published both animal
and clinical studies in which they report encouraging results in treating
arsenic-poisoned mice and humans with a "potentized homeopathic remedy," namely Arsenicum album. If these results are substantiated by others,
it could represent an important development in the fight to save the health
of people forced to drink arsenic-contaminated water. Some scientists, however, urge caution in interpreting the results of these studies.[52]

Arsenic in Contemporary Folk Remedies and Patent Medicine

Arsenic is a common ingredient in various folk remedies and patent medicines, especially those from Asia. In a study carried out by the California
Department of Health Services in 1996, for example, arsenic was found as
an undeclared ingredient in 36 out of 260 Asian patent medicines collected
from California retail herbal stores. The average concentration of arsenic in
these remedies was 14,553 parts per million, many times the recommended
level of under 30 parts per million. In another study in 2008, researchers
focused on Ayurvedic medicines manufactured in the United States and
India and sold via the Internet. They found that about 21 percent of them
contained lead, mercury, or arsenic in amounts exceeding acceptable daily
metal intake levels, although arsenic was the least common of the metals
found in this sample. A British study in 2002 analyzed the published literature on the heavy-metal content of traditional Indian remedies and reported
that 41 percent of them had been shown to contain significant amounts of
arsenic. An Australian investigation in 2007 determined that about 5 percent
of 247 traditional Chinese medicines analyzed contained arsenic, and a Dutch
study in 2010 reported that 26 of 292 Asian herbal preparations examined
contained arsenic significantly above the safety limit for this substance.[53]

　　Not surprisingly, there have been reported cases of poisoning as a result
of taking some of these medicines. For example, as early as 1975, a paper in
the *Medical Journal of Australia* reported that 64 percent of 74 cases of chronic
arsenic poisoning over a fifteen-month period in Singapore were found to
be caused by a local anti-asthmatic herbal preparation containing 12,000
parts per million of inorganic arsenic sulfide. The other patients in this group

were poisoned by six other brands of Chinese herbal remedies containing high concentrations of inorganic arsenic. Some of the patients involved had been taking these preparations for as long as fifteen years. The poisoning affected the skin, nervous system, gastrointestinal system, and blood in various patients, including six cases of skin malignancies.[54]

Various other studies have demonstrated the potential toxic effects of certain traditional medicines. Another report from Singapore in 1998 discussed seventeen cases of patients with skin lesions related to chronic arsenic poisoning caused by Chinese proprietary medicines known to contain inorganic arsenic. Researchers in London described in a 1993 paper two cases of heavy metal intoxication resulting from ingestion of Indian ethnic remedies. The users had received the medicines, which were found to contain toxic amounts of mercury and arsenic, from a hakim, an Indian ethnic practitioner, for the treatment of eczema.[55]

The use of traditional Asian medicines has been increasing in popularity, even among Western populations. These products, like other herbal remedies and supplements, are not strictly regulated in many countries, including the United States, and they are readily available without prescription. The presence of heavy metals is generally not indicated on the labels of these products. The extent of the health problem involved is unclear, however, as most of the data concerning these products is anecdotal and insufficient to obtain reliable statistics on use and incidence of toxic reactions. Some health professionals have argued, however, that better ways should be found to maximize consumer safety.

The problem presented by these medicines illustrates once more one of the themes of this book, that arsenic is a double-edged sword and that there is a fine line between the two sides. The properties that make arsenic useful as a medicine, and for certain other uses such as a pesticide and preservative, are the same properties that make it dangerous as a poison. Arsenic can kill cancer cells but at the same time can damage the human cells of the recipient of the medicine. Arsenic can eliminate pests such as rats and insects, but its use as a pesticide and preservative can also lead to environmental problems. As this book has documented, arsenic has proved useful over the ages for an amazing number and varieties of purposes. When all is said and done, however, it will still mostly be thought of as the King of Poisons.

Suggested Further Readings

There is an extensive literature on arsenic and its history. The chapter notes in this volume provide hundred of references to works on various aspects of the subject. The following selected list, however, can provide an entry into this large and diverse body of literature for the reader interested in learning more about the history of arsenic.

Books

Burney, Ian. *Poison, Detection, and the Victorian Imagination*. Manchester, UK: Manchester University Press, 2006.

Committee on Medical and Biologic Effects of Environmental Pollution. *Arsenic*. Washington, DC: National Academy of Sciences, 1977.

Cullen, William R. *Is Arsenic an Aphrodisiac: The Sociochemistry of an Element*. Cambridge, UK: RSC Publishing, 2008.

Emsley, John. *The Elements of Murder: A History of Poison*. New York: Oxford University Press, 2005.

Meharg, Andrew A. *Venomous Earth: How Arsenic Caused the World's Worst Mass Poisoning*. Houndmills, UK: Macmillan, 2005.

Watson, Katherine. *Poisoned Lives: English Poisoners and Their Victims*. London: Hambledon and London, 2004.

Whorton, James C. *The Arsenic Century: How Victorian Britain Was Poisoned at Home, Work, and Play*. New York: Oxford University Press, 2010.

Articles

Bartrip, P. W. J. "'A Pennuth of Arsenic for Rat Poison': The Arsenic Act of 1851 and the Prevention of Secret Poisoning." *Medical History* 36 (1992): 53–69.

Bartrip, P. W. J. "How Green Was My Valence?: Environmental Arsenic Poisoning and the Victorian Domestic Ideal." *English Historical Review* 109 (1994): 891–913.

Bentley, Ronald, and Thomas G. Chasteen. "Arsenic Curiosa and Humanity." *Chemical Educator* 7 (2002): 51–60.

Doyle, Derek. "Notoriety to Respectability: A Short History of Arsenic Prior to Its Present Day Use in Haematology." *British Journal of Haematology* 1445 (2009): 309–17.

Haller Jr., John S. "*Therapeutic Mule*: The Use of Arsenic in the Nineteenth-Century Materia Medica." *Pharmacy in History* 17 (1975): 87–100.

Joliffe, D. M. "A History of the Use of Arsenicals in Man." *Journal of the Royal Society of Medicine* 86 (1993): 287–89.

Mandal, Badal Kumar, and Kazuo T. Suzuki. "Arsenic Round the World: A Review." *Talanta* 58 (2002): 201–35.

Scheindlin, Stanley. "The Duplicitous Nature of Inorganic Arsenic." *Molecular Interventions* 5, no. 2 (April 2005): 60–64.

Winn, Kenneth H. "Arsenic Eaters in the Nineteenth Century." *Gateway* 29 (2009): 74–83.

Notes

Introduction

1. John Emsley, *The Elements of Murder: A History of Poison* (New York: Oxford University Press, 2005), 93.

2. William R. Cullen, *Is Arsenic an Aphrodisiac? The Sociochemistry of an Element* (Cambridge, UK: RSC Publishing, 2008), 287.

3. Felisa Wolfe-Simon et al., "A Bacterium That Can Grow by Using Arsenic Instead of Phosphorus," *Science* 332 (2011): 1163–66 . For critiques of this work, see the comments published in *Science* 332 (2011): 1149. On the recent criticism in *Science*, see Marc Kaufman, "Journal Science Retreats from Controversial Arsenic Paper," *Washington Post*, July 9, 2012.

1. King of Poisons: Arsenic and Murder

1. Andrew A. Meharg, *Venomous Earth: How Arsenic Caused the World's Worst Mass Poisoning* (Houndmills, UK: Macmillan, 2005), 41; William R. Cullen, *Is Arsenic an Aphrodisiac?*, 167; John Harris Trestrail III, *Criminal Poisoning: Investigational Guide for Law Enforcement, Toxicologists, Forensic Scientists, and Attorneys*, 2nd ed. (Totowa, NJ: Humana, 2007), 1–6; John Emsley, *The Elements of Murder*, 141.

2. Cullen, *Is Arsenic an Aphrodisiac?*, 168–69; Trestrail, *Criminal Poisoning*, 6–7.

3. Cullen, *Is Arsenic an Aphrodisiac?*, 168; Trestrail, *Criminal Poisoning*, 7. For a challenge to the traditional view of Catherine, see N. M. Sutherland, "Catherine de Medici: The Legend of the Wicked Italian Queen," *Sixteenth Century Journal* 9 (1978): 45–56.

4. Anne Somerset, *The Affair of the Poisons: Murder, Infanticide and Satanism in the Court of Louis XIV* (New York: St. Martin's, 2003).

5. Ian Burney, *Poison, Detection, and the Victorian Imagination* (Manchester, England: Manchester University Press, 2006), 19; Cullen, *Is Arsenic an Aphrodisiac?*, 169; Frank McLynn, *Crime and Punishment in Eighteenth-Century England* (London: Routledge, 1989), 119.

6. Burney, *Poison Detection*, 19–20; Katherine Watson, *Poisoned Lives: English Poisoners and Their Victims* (London: Hambledon Continuum, 2004), 32–33. The quotation is on page 32.

7. Watson, *Poisoned Lives*, 32–38.

8. Ibid., xii–xiii.

9. Watson, *Poisoned Lives*, 45; Burney, *Poison Detection*, 21.

10. Watson, *Poisoned Lives*, 2–3, 7–11.

11. Ibid., 3–5; Cullen, *Arsenic*, 172.

12. Watson, *Poisoned Lives*, 17–19; Cullen, *Is Arsenic an Aphrodisiac?*, 173; Burney, *Poison Detection*, 97–100. For a detailed account of the development of chemical tests for arsenic, see Robert H. Goldsmith, "The Search for Arsenic," in *More Chemistry and Crime: From Marsh Arsenic Test to DNA Profile*, eds. Samuel M. Gerber and Richard Saferstein (Washington, DC: American Chemical Society, 1997), 149–68.

13. Cullen, *Is Arsenic an Aphrodisiac?*, 174–76.

14. Ibid., 174; Watson, *Poisoned Lives*, 19.

15. Peter Bartrip, "A 'Pennurth of Arsenic for Rat Poison': The Arsenic Act, 1851 and the Prevention of Secret Poisoning," *Medical History* 36 (1992): 53–69; Watson, *Poisoned Lives*, 42–44; Leslie G. Matthews, *History of Pharmacy in Britain* (Edinburgh: E. & S. Livingstone, 1962), 119–20, 369–70.

16. Stuart Anderson, ed., *Making Medicines: A Brief History of Pharmacy and Pharmaceuticals* (London: Pharmaceutical Press, 2005), 101–3; Matthews, *History of Pharmacy*, 134–36; Watson, *Poisoned Lives*, 43–44; Hugh N. Linstead, *Poisons Law* (London: Pharmaceutical Press, 1936), 1–18.

17. M. I. Wilbert, "The Evolution of Laws Regulating the Sale and Use of Poisons," *Journal of the American Pharmaceutical Association* 1 (1912): 1259–61; Martin I. Wilbert, "Sale and Use of Poison," *Public Health Reports* 29 (1914): 3027–30.

18. Wilbert, "Sale and Use," 3029.

19. The discussion of this case is based on Bruce Chadwick, *I Am Murdered: George Wythe, Thomas Jefferson, and the Killing That Shocked a New Nation* (Hoboken, NJ: John Wiley and Sons, 2009).

20. The discussion of this case is based largely on Douglas MacGowan, *The Strange Affair of Madeleine Smith: Victorian Scotland's Trial of the Century* (Edinburgh: Mercat, 2007); Jimmy Powdrell Campbell, *A Scottish Murder: Rewriting the Madeleine Smith Story* (Stroud, England: Tempus, 2007); and H. B. Irving, ed., *Trial of Mrs. Maybrick*, 2nd ed., 2nd impression (Edinburgh: William Hodge, 1927).

21. For a detailed discussion of the extensive literature on the Smith case, see MacGowan, *Strange Affair*, 142–49.

22. Campbell, *Scottish Murder*.

23. The discussion of this case is based largely on Trevor L. Christie, *Etched in Arsenic: A New Study of the Maybrick Case* (London: George G. Harrap, 1969); Victoria Blake, *Mrs. Maybrick* (Kew: National Archives, 2008); and Emsley, *Elements of Murder*, 71–93.

24. Christie, *Etched in Arsenic*, 265–74; Blake, *Mrs. Maybrick*, 102–8.

25. Emsley, *Elements of Murder*, 171–93.

26. The discussion of this case is based largely on Filson Young, ed., *Trial of the Seddons* (Edinburgh: William Hodge, 1914) and Edgar Wallace, "The Trial of the

Seddons," in *Solved: Famous Mystery Writers on Classic True-Crime Cases*, ed. Richard Glyn Jones (New York: Peter Bedrick Books, 1987), 195–211.

27. The discussion of this case is based largely on Robin Odell, *Exhumation of a Murder: The Life and Trial of Major Armstrong* (New York: St. Martin's, 1989); Frank Jones, *Beyond Suspicion: True Stories of Unexpected Killers* (Toronto: Key Porter Books, 1992), 53–84; and Filson Young, ed., *Trial of Herbert Rowse Armstrong*, reprint edition (n.p.: Hesperides Press, 2008).

28. The discussion of this case is based largely on Richard Whittington-Egan, *The Riddle of Birdhurst Rise: The Croydon Poisoning Mystery* (London: Penguin Books, 1988) and Jean Graham Hall and Gordon Smith, *The Croydon Arsenic Mystery* (Chichester: Barry Rose Law Publishers, 1999).

29. The discussion of this case is based largely on Béla Bodó, "The Poisoning Women of Tiszazug," *Journal of Family History* 27 (2002): 40–59 and Ferenc Gyorgyey, "Arsenic and No Lace," *Caduceus* 3 (1987): 41–64.

30. Quoted in English translation in Gyorgyey, "Arsenic," 54.

31. Quoted in English translation in ibid., 48.

32. Bodó, "Poisoning Women," 43.

33. Robert Horton, "Food for Thought," *Film Comment* 44, no. 1 (January–February, 2008): 32–34; Derek Elley, "Hukkle," *Variety*, February 18–24, 2002, 41; Sheila Johnston, "Hukkle," October 31, 2002, http://www.screendaily.com/hukkle /4011020.article; Andrew Higgins, "Hungarian Town with a Toxic Past Wants to Cash In," *Wall Street Journal* (Eastern Edition), May 20, 2004.

34. "Arsenic and No Lace: The Bizarre Tale of a Philadelphia Murder Ring," *Pennsylvania History* 67 (2000): 397–414.

35. One example in the period after World War II is Velma Barfield of North Carolina, who confessed in 1978 to murdering four people with arsenic. She was executed by lethal injection on November 2, 1984, the first woman to die by this method. For more on Barfield, see Jerry Bledsoe, *Death Sentence: The True Story of Velma Barfield's Life, Crimes and Execution* (New York: Dutton, 1998).

36. The discussion of this case is based largely on Amanda Lamb, *Deadly Dose: The Untold Story of a Homicide Investigator's Crusade for Truth and Justice* (New York: Berkley Books, 2008).

37. The discussion of this case is based largely on Christine Ellen Young, *A Bitter Brew: Faith, Power, and Poison in a Small New England Town* (New York: Berkley Books, 2005).

38. Quoted in ibid., 229.

39. Pam Bellick, "Poisonings at Church Are Termed Retaliation," *New York Times*, April 19, 2006.

40. Renee Ordway, "Women's Death Reminder of Toll from Poisonings," *Bangor Daily News*, April 10, 2009; "*Mystery ER* episode descriptions," Discovery Health Channel, http://health.discovery.com/tv/mystery-er/episode-guide.html.

41. The discussion of arsenic in chemical warfare is based largely on Joel A. Velinsky, *Dew of Death: The Story of Lewisite, America's World War I Weapon of Mass Destruction* (Bloomington: Indiana University Press, 2005); Cullen, *Is Arsenic an Aphrodisiac?*, 215–86; Joel A. Velinsky and Pandy R. Sinish, "The Dew of Death,"

Bulletin of the Atomic Scientists 60, no. 2 (March/April, 2004): 54–60; Gilbert F. Whittemore Jr., "World War I, Gas Research, and the Ideals of American Chemists," *Social Studies of Science* 5 (1975): 135–63.

42. Warren E. Leary, "U.S. to Compensate Ex-G.I.'s Exposed to Poison Gases," *New York Times*, January 7, 1993.

43. Pandy R. Sinish and Joel A. Vilensky, "WMDs in Our Backyards," *Earth Island Journal* 19, no. 4 (Winter 2005): 31–34.

2. Poison in the Plot: Arsenic in Fiction

1. John Harris Trestrail III, *Criminal Poisoning: Investigational Guide for Law Enforcement, Toxicologists, Forensic Scientists, and Attorneys*, 2nd ed. (Totowa, NJ: Humana, 2007), 97–100.

2. On the history of detective fiction, see Charles J. Rzepka, *Detective Fiction* (Cambridge, England: Polity, 2005) and A. Craig Bell, "The Rise and Fall of the Detective Novel," *Contemporary Review* 272 (1998): 196–200. The works of Poe, Doyle, Dickens, and Collins have been issued in numerous editions, so no specific editions are cited here except in the case of quotations.

3. Quoted in David Deirdre, ed., *The Cambridge Companion to the Victorian Novel* (Cambridge: Cambridge University Press, 2001), 179.

4. Jenny Bourne Taylor, "Introduction," in Wilkie Collins, *The Law and the Lady* (Oxford: Oxford University Press, 2008), xix–xx.

5. A copy of the story may be found in R. Austin Freeman, *The Best Dr. Thorndyke Stories* (New York: Dover Publications, 1973). The introduction to this volume by E. F. Bleiler (v–ix) provides brief information on Freeman and the Thorndyke character.

6. R. Austin Freeman, *As a Thief in the Night* (North Yorkshire, England: House of Stratus, 2001), 71.

7. James C. Whorton, *The Arsenic Century: How Victorian Britain was Poisoned at Home, Work, and Play* (Oxford: Oxford University Press, 2010), 169–76.

8. Phoebe Atwood Taylor, *Death Lights a Candle* (Woodstock, VT: Foul Plays, 1989).

9. Dashiell Hammett, "Fly Paper," *Black Mask* 12, no. 6 (August 1929): 7–26.

10. Erle Stanley Gardner, *The Case of the Drowsy Mosquito* (New York: Pocket Books, 1966).

11. Paul Doherty, *The Queen of the Night* (London: Headline, 2006). The quotations from the novel are on pages 385 and 54. The author's note is on 397–400.

12. Cullen, *Is Arsenic an Aphrodisiac?*, 81–84; John L. Konefes and Michael K. McGee, "Old Cemeteries, Arsenic, and Health Safety," *Cultural Resources Management* 19, no. 10 (1996): 15–18.

13. Terri Blackstock, *Shadow of Doubt* (Grand Rapids, MI: Zondervan, 1998).

14. Bertram Atkey, *Arsenic and Gold* (Philadelphia: Penn Publishing, 1939); Sharyn McCrumb, *If I'd Killed Him When I Met Him* (New York: Ballantine Books, 1995); Hailey Lind, *Arsenic and Old Paint* (Palo Alto, CA: Perseverance, 2010).

15. Michael C. Gerald, *The Poisonous Pen of Agatha Christie* (Austin: University of Texas Press, 1993), viii.

16. Ibid., 136.

17. For biographical information on Christie, see Laura Thompson, *Agatha Christie: An English Mystery* (London: Headline, 2008). There have been so many published editions of Christie's novels and stories and they are so widely available that I have not cited any specific editions.

18. Thompson, *Christie*, 103–4.

19. Gerald, *Poisonous Pen*, 6.

20. There have been several biographies of Sayers, the most recent of which is Barbara Reynolds, *Dorothy L. Sayers: Her Life and Soul* (London: Hodder and Stoughton, 1993; revised editions in 1998 and 2002).

21. Fredrick Accum, *A Treatise on Adulterations of Food, and Culinary Poisons* (London: Longman, Hurst, Rees, Orme, and Brown, 1820), vii.

22. Dorothy L. Sayers, *Strong Poison* (Cleveland: World Publishing Company, 1945), 245–46.

23. A. E. Housman, *A Shropshire Lad* (London: Grant Richards, 1908), 100.

24. Dorothy L. Sayers, "Suspicion," in *Handbook for Poisoners: A Collection of Great Poison Stories*, ed. Raymond T. Bond (New York: Collier Books, 1962), 79–95. The quotation is on page 95.

25. Geoffrey Chaucer, *The Riverside Chaucer*, new edition (Oxford, England: Oxford University Press, 2008), 273.

26. Ben Johnson, *The Alchemist*, edited by H. C. Hart (London: De La More, 1903), 47, 209. Meharg, *Venomous Earth*, 49–50, also translates "Zernich" as arsenic but does not give a source for this interpretation.

27. Whorton, *Arsenic Century*, 214–18.

28. Beth Sutton-Ramspeck, *The Literary Housekeeping of Mary Ward, Sarah Grand, and Charlotte Perkins Gilman* (Athens: Ohio University Press, 2004), 123–25.

29. See Catherine J. Golden, ed., *Charlotte Perkins Gilman's* The Yellow Wall-Paper: *A Sourcebook and Critical Edition* (New York: Routledge, 2004) for a broad sampling of various views of Gilman's story.

30. On Flaubert and the controversy over *Madame Bovary*, see Francis Steegmuller, *Flaubert and Madame Bovary: A Double Portrait* (New York: Viking Press, 1939) and Geoffrey Wall, *Flaubert: A Life* (London: Faber and Faber, 2001).

31. Gustave Flaubert, *Madame Bovary*, translated by Lowell Blair (New York: Bantam, 2005), 312.

32. Joseph Kesselring, *Arsenic and Old Lace* (New York: Dramatists Play Service, 1995), 26.

33. M. William Phelps, *The Devil's Rooming House: The True Story of America's Deadliest Female Serial Killer* (Guilford, CT: Lyons Press, 2010).

34. Charles Busch, *Die, Mommy, Die!* (New York: Samuel French, 2005).

35. William Faulkner, "A Rose for Emily," in *The Portable Faulkner*, revised and expanded edition, ed. Malcolm Cowley (New York: Viking, 1967), 433–44. The quotation is on page 443–44.

36. Shirley Jackson, *We Have Always Lived in the Castle* (New York: Viking, 1962).

37. Robert Goolrick, *A Reliable Wife* (Chapel Hill, NC: Algonquin Books, 2009), 201.

38. On the Peales, see Lillian B. Miller, ed., *The Peale Family: Creation of a Legacy 1770–1870* (New York: Abbeville, 1996).

39. Mary E. Lyons, *The Poison Place* (New York: Atheneum Books for Young Readers, 1997), 158–59.

40. Niamh Russell, "The Benefits of Arsenic," in *Harlem River Blues and Other Stories: Fish Anthology 2008*, ed. Jack Hawson (County Cork, Ireland: Fish, 2008), 61–62. The quotation is on page 61.

3. Hazards on the Job: Arsenic in the Workplace

1. Jerome O. Nriagu, "Arsenic Poisoning Through the Ages," in *Environmental Chemistry of Arsenic*, ed. William T. Frankenberger Jr. (New York: Marcel Dekker, 2002), 1–26. The quotation is on page 2.

2. George Rosen, *The History of Miners' Diseases: A Medical and Social Interpretation* (New York: Schuman's, 1943), 36–88. The quotation is on page 76.

3. Bernardino Ramazzini, *A Treatise on the Diseases of Tradesmen* (London: A. Bell, 1705), 61.

4. Ibid., 11, 26–27. On Ramazzini's discussion of the diseases of miners, see also Rosen, *Miners' Diseases*, 108–20.

5. Rosen, *Miners' Diseases*, 123–24, 192–93.

6. Charles Turner Thackrah, *The Effects of Arts, Trades, and Professions, and of Civic States and Habits of Living, on Health and Longevity*, 2nd ed. (London: Longman, Rees, Orme, Brown, Green and Longman, 1832), 92.

7. Meharg, *Venomous Earth*, 133.

8. Ibid., 135.

9. M. Harper, "Occupational Health Aspects of the Arsenic Extractive Industry in Britain, 1868–1925," *British Journal of Industrial Medicine* 45 (1988): 602–5. The quotation is on page 605.

10. N. Ishinishi et al., "Outbreak of Chronic Arsenic Poisoning among Retired Workers from an Arsenic Mine in Japan," *Environmental Health Perspectives* 19 (1977): 121–25; Marianne Sullivan, "Contested Science and Exposed Workers: ASARCO and the Occupational Standard for Inorganic Arsenic," *Public Health Reports* 122 (2007): 541–47; Jay H. Lubin et al., "Respiratory Cancer and Inhaled Inorganic Arsenic in Copper Smelter Workers: A Linear Relationship with Cumulative Exposure that Increases with Concentration," *Environmental Health Perspectives* 116 (2008): 1661–65. The quotation is on page 1665. For other examples, see Cullen, *Is Arsenic an Aphrodisiac?*, 313–25.

11. The discussion of arsenic poisoning in the artificial flower industry is based on Whorton, *Arsenic Century*, 183–86, and P. W. J. Bartrip, *The Home Office and the Dangerous Trades: Regulating Occupational Disease in Victorian and Edwardian Britain* (Amsterdam: Rodopi, 2002), 140–48.

12. Bartrip, *Dangerous Trades*, 146.

13. Ibid., 151.

14. The discussion of this investigation is based on ibid., 148–52.

15. Ibid., 149.

16. Ibid., 149.

17. Ibid., 152.

18. "The Manufacture of Mineral Pigments," *British Medical Journal* 1 (1893): 753–54. The quotation is on page 753.

19. Ramazzini, *Diseases of Tradesmen*, 39–43. The quotation is on page 41.

20. Thackrah, *Effects of Arts*, 106–9.

21. George Rosen, "Occupational Health Problems of English Painters and Varnishers in 1825," *British Journal of Industrial Medicine* 10 (1953): 195–99.

22. Vincent Daniels and Bridget Leach, "The Occurrence and Alteration of Realgar on Ancient Egyptian Papyri," *Studies in Conservation* 49 (2004): 73–84; William Foster, "Chemistry and Grecian Archaeology," *Journal of Chemical Education* 10 (1933): 270–77; Nancy Purinton and Mark Watters, "A Study of the Materials Used by Medieval Persian Painters," *Journal of the American Institute for Conservation* 30 (1991): 125–44; Alicia Seldes et al., "Green, Yellow, and Red Pigments in South American Painting, 1610–1780," *Journal of the American Institute for Conservation* 41 (2002): 225–42; Lisbet Milling Pedersen and Henrik Permin, "Rheumatic Disease, Heavy-Metal Pigments, and the Great Masters," *Lancet* 1 (1988): 1267–69; and Janice H. Carlson and John Krill, "Pigment Analysis in Early American Watercolors and Fraktur," *Journal of the American Institute for Conservation* 18 (1978): 19–32.

23. On the history of taxidermy, see Stephen T. Asma, *Stuffed Animals and Pickled Heads: The Culture and Evolution of Natural History Museums* (Oxford, England: Oxford University Press, 2001); Melissa Milgrom, *Still Life: Adventures in Taxidermy* (Boston: Houghton Mifflin Harcourt, 2010); Christopher Frost, *A History of British Taxidermy* (Long Melford, England: C. Frost, 1987); and Pat Morris, *A History of Taxidermy: Art, Science and Bad Taste* (Ascot, England: MGM Publishing, 2010).

24. Paul Lawrence Farber, "The Development of Taxidermy and the History of Ornithology," *Isis* 68 (1977): 550–66; Fernando Marte, Amadine Péquignot, and David W. Von Endt, "Arsenic in Taxidermy Collections: History, Detection, and Management," *Collection Forum* 21 (2006): 143–50.

25. C. A. Walker, "Hints on Taxidermy," *American Naturalist* 3 (1869): 136–46, 189–201.

26. Asma, *Stuffed Animals*, 22; Mark V. Barrow Jr., "The Specimen Dealer: Entrepreneurial Natural History in America's Gilded Age," *Journal of the History of Biology* 33 (2000): 493–534.

27. Marte, Péquignot, and Von Endt, "Arsenic in Taxidermy;" Lisa Goldberg, "A History of Pest Control Measures in the Anthropology Collections, National Museum of Natural History, Smithsonian Institution," *Journal of the American Institute for Conservation* 35 (1996): 23–43.

28. Cullen, *Is Arsenic an Aphrodisiac?*, 85.

29. J. N. Gannal, *History of Embalming, and of Preparations in Anatomy, Pathology and Natural History; Including an Account of a New Process for Embalming*, translated by R. Harlan (Philadelphia: Judah Dobson, 1840), 169.

30. Gunde E. Jensen and Inge L. B. Olsen, "Occupational Exposure to Inorganic Arsenic in Wood Workers and Taxidermists — Air Sampling and Biological Monitoring," *Journal of Environmental Science and Health, Part A* 30 (1995): 921–38; George M. Kober and William C. Hanson, eds., *Diseases of Occupation and Vocational Hygiene* (Philadelphia: P. Blakiston's Son, 1916), 5–6; William N. Rom, ed., *Environmental and Occupational Medicine*, 4th ed. (Philadelphia: Lippincott Williams and Wilkins, 2007), 1007.

31. Pat Morris, "Stuffing for Longevity," *New Scientist* 95 (1982): 575.

32. Melissa Milgrom, *Still Life: Adventures in Taxidermy* (Boston: Houghton Mifflin Harcourt, 2010), 23–24.

33. Phoebe Lloyd and Gordon Bendersky, "Arsenic, An Old Case: The Chronic Heavy Metal Poisoning of Raphaelle Peale (1774–1825)," *Perspectives in Biology and Medicine* 36 (1993): 654–65. The quotation is on page 655.

34. William H. Honan, "Suspicions of Hatred in a Family of Artists," *New York Times*, July 5, 1993.

35. Phoebe Lloyd, "Invisible Killers: Heavy Metals, Saturnine Envy, and the Tragic Death of Raphaelle Peale," *Transactions and Studies of the College of Physicians of Philadelphia* 16 (1994): 83–99; Lillian B. Miller, "History and the Peales," *Transactions and Studies*, 101–6.

36. On the early history of embalming, see R. G. Meyer, *Embalming: History, Theory, and Practice*, 4th ed. (New York: McGraw Hill, 2005); Dániel Margócsy, "Advertising Cadavers in the Republic of Letters: Anatomical Publications in the Early Modern Netherlands," *British Journal of the History of Science* 42 (2009): 187–210; Pascale Trompette and Mélanie Lemonnier, "Funeral Embalming: The Transformation of a Medical Innovation," *Science Studies* 22 (2009): 9–30; Jolene Zigarovich, "Preserved Remains: Embalming Practices in Eighteenth-Century England," *Eighteenth-Century Life* 33 (2009): 65–104.

37. Trompette and Lemonnier, "Funeral Embalming," 12.

38. This discussion of the history of embalming is based on Trompette and Lemonier, "Funeral Embalming"; Cullen, *Is Arsenic an Aphrodisiac?*, 81–84; M. L. Ajmani, *Embalming: Principles and Legal Aspects* (New Delhi: Jaypee Brothers, 1998), 24–31; and Arthur C. Aufderhede, *The Scientific Study of Mummies* (Cambridge, England: Cambridge University Press, 2003), 68–69.

39. Trompette and Lemonier, "Funeral Embalming," 15.

40. Cullen, *Is Arsenic an Aphrodisiac?*, 83.

41. Christine Quigley, *Modern Mummies: The Preservation of the Human Body in the Twentieth Century* (Jefferson, NC: McFarland, 1998), 60–64.

42. Gannal, *History of Embalming*, 210–11.

43. Ajmani, *Embalming*, 26; Cullen, *Is Arsenic an Aphrodisiac?*, 82.

44. Carl Lewis Barnes, *The Art and Science of Embalming* (Chicago: Trade Periodical Company, 1898).

45. See, for example, John L. Konefes and Michael K. McGee, "Old Cemeteries, Arsenic, and Health Safety," *Cultural Resource Management* 19, no. 10 (1996): 15–18; Mark Harris, *Grave Matters: A Journey through the Modern Funeral Industry to a National Way of Burying* (New York: Scribner, 2007), 38; and Clifton D. Bryant,

Handbook of Death and Dying, vol. 1 (Thousand Oaks, CA: Sage Publications, 2003), 541.

46. See, for example, Frederick Peterson and Walter S. Haines, eds., *A Textbook of Legal Medicine and Toxicology*, vol. 2 (Philadelphia: W. B. Saunders, 1904), 430, 708, 721; Justin Herold, *A Manual of Legal Medicine* (Philadelphia: J. B. Lippincott, 1898), 140–42; and Thomas M. Durell, "A Protest Against Embalming," *Boston Medical and Surgical Journal* 122 (1890): 544–55.

47. Durell, "Protest Against Embalming," 545.

48. Ajmani, *Embalming: Principles*, 47; Aufderhede, *Study of Mummies*, 69; Bryant, *Handbook of Death*, 541.

49. Quigley, *Modern Mummies*, 6; Patricia A. Dempsey, George R. Kelder, Jr., and Michael Mittenzwei, "The Future of Formaldehyde: Risks, Regulations, Protections and Alternatives," *The Forum* 75, no. 3 (January 2009): 22–28.

50. Merrill Singer et al., "Dust in the Wind: The Growing Use of Embalming Fluid Among Youth in Hartford, CT," *Substance Use and Misuse* 40 (2005): 1035–50.

51. Whorton, *Arsenic Century*, 289–90.

52. Konefes and McGee, "Old Cemeteries," 17.

53. Whorton, *Arsenic Century*, 311–316. The quotation is on page 312.

54. Ibid., 312–13.

55. Lawrence T. Fairhall, *Industrial Toxicology*, 2nd ed. (Baltimore: Williams and Wilkins, 1957), 18.

56. James Whorton, *Before Silent Spring: Pesticides and Public Health in Pre-DDT America* (Princeton, NJ: Princeton University Press, 1974); Radoslaw Spiewak, "Pesticides as a Cause of Occupational Skin Diseases in Farmers," *Annals of Agriculture and Environmental Medicine* 8 (2001): 1–5; Gunnar F. Nordberg, Bruce A. Fowler, Monica Nordberg, and Lars Friberg, *Handbook on the Toxicology of Metals*, 3rd ed. (Burlington, MA: Academic, 2007), 183; Hyman J. Zimmerman, *Hepatotoxicity: The Adverse Effects of Drugs and Other Chemicals on the Liver*, 2nd ed. (Philadelphia: Lippincott Williams and Wilkins, 199), 372–73; Susan W. Lanman, "Colour in the Garden: 'Malignant Magenta,'" *Garden History* 28 (2000): 209–21; M. D. Kipling, "Arsenic," in *Environment and Man*, vol. 6: *The Chemical Environment* (New York: Academic, 1977), 93–120; K. Rosenman, "Occupational Heart Disease," in *Environmental and Occupational Medicine*, ed. W. Rom and S. Markowitz, 4th ed. (Philadelphia: Lippincott, Williams and Wilkins, 2007), 688.

57. Jensen and Olsen, "Occupational Exposure"; James Huff, "Sawmill Chemicals and Carcinogenesis," *Environmental Health Perspectives* 109 (2001): 209–12; "Chromated Copper Arsenate (CCA)," Environmental Protection Agency, http://www.epa.gov/oppad001/reregistration/cca/index.htm#general.

58. John B. Sullivan Jr. and Gary R. Krieger, eds., *Clinical Environmental Health and Toxic Exposures*, 2nd ed. (Philadelphia: Lippincott, Williams and Wilkins, 2001), 864.

4. The Ubiquitous Element: Arsenic in the Environment

1. Whorton, *Arsenic Century*, x.

2. P. W. J. Bartrip, "How Green was My Valance?: Environmental Arsenic Poisoning and the Victorian Domestic Ideal," *English Historical Review* 109 (1994): 891–913. The quotation is on page 895.

3. Whorton, *Arsenic Century*, xi.

4. Ibid., 176–77; Bartrip, "How Green," 895–96.

5. Bartip, "How Green," 895; Whorton, *Arsenic Century*, 177–78.

6. Malcolm Morris, "Arsenic in Wall-Papers and Paints," in *Our Homes and How to Make Them Healthy*, ed. Shirley Foster Murphy (London: Cassell, 1883), 365–72; J. K. Haywood and H. J. Warner, *Arsenic in Papers and Fabric* (Washington, DC: Government Printing Office, 1904), 14–20.

7. Meharg, *Venomous Earth*, 85–86. The quotation from *The Times* is on page 86.

8. Morris, "Arsenic in Wall-Papers," 366; Whorton, *Arsenic Century*, 194–95; Meharg, *Venomous Earth*, 89.

9. Bartrip, "How Green," 897–98. The quotation is on page 898.

10. William R. Cullen and Ronald Bentley, "The Toxicity of Trimethylarsine: An Urban Myth," *Journal of Environmental Monitoring* 7 (2005): 11–15; Bartrip, "How Green," 899; Whorton, *Arsenic Century*, 206–7.

11. Bartrip, "How Green," 900; Whorton, *Arsenic Century*, 207; William E. Rice, "Case of Poisoning by Arsenic in Wall-Paper," *Boston Medical and Surgical Journal* 69 (1863): 297.

12. Bartrip, "How Green," 901; Whorton, *Arsenic Century*, 208–9.

13. Fiona MacCarthy, "Morris, William," *Oxford Dictionary of National Biography* 39 (2004): 317–24; Andrew Meharg, "The Arsenic Green," *Nature* 423 (2003): 688 (source of quotation); Meharg, *Venemous Earth*, 77–78.

14. The quotations are taken from Morris's letters as reproduced in Meharg, *Venomous Earth*, 82.

15. Whorton, *Arsenic Century*, 210–12. The quotation is on page 212.

16. Bartrip, "How Green," 906–9. The correspondence received from various countries by the British government was reprinted in *Correspondence Reflecting the Presence of Arsenic and Other Poisonous Pigments in Wall-papers and Textile Fabrics* (London: Harrison and Sons, 1883).

17. See, e.g., J. J. Putnam, "On the Character and Injuriousness of Arsenic as a Domestic Poison," *Journal of the American Medical Association* 16 (1891): 778–81; W. B. Hills, "Detection of Arsenic in Wall Paper," *Boston Medical and Surgical Journal* 104 (1881): 29; "Arsenic in Common Use," *New York Times*, December 14, 1884; "Arsenic in Wallpaper," *New York Times*, February 11, 1892.

18. Frank W. Draper, "Arsenic in Certain Green Colors," in *Third Annual Report of the State Board of Health of Massachusetts* (Boston: Wright and Potter, 1872), 17–57. The quotation is on page 33.

19. Ibid., 33, 57. The quotation is on page 57.

20. George P. Merk, "Robert C. Kedzie, Michigan's Nineteenth Century Consumer Activist," *Michigan History* 73 (1989): 16–23; Robert E. Mosher and G. Elaine Beane, "The Beginning of Public Health in Michigan: Michigan State Board of Health Reports, 1873-1900," *Michigan Journal of Public Health* 2 (2008): 10–20.

21. R. C. Kedzie, *Shadows from the Walls of Death* (Lansing, MI: State Board of Health of Michigan, 1874), 1–8. The quotations are on page 5. A copy of the book is in the History of Medicine Division of the National Library of Medicine.

22. Edward S. Wood, *Arsenic as a Domestic Poison* (Boston: Massachusetts State Board of Health, Lunacy and Charity, 1885).

23. Ibid., 5.

24. Bartrip, "How Green," 911–12.

25. Whorton, *Arsenic Century*, 225; Hayward and Warner, *Arsenic in Paper*; Putnam, "On the Character."

26. Cullen, *Is Arsenic an Aphrodisiac?*, 109–10.

27. Ibid., 110–11.

28. Ibid., 111, 118; Cullen and Bentley, "The Toxicity of Trimethylarsine," 11–15.

29. Haywood and Warner, *Arsenic in Paper*, 13.

30. Cullen, *Is Arsenic an Aphrodisiac?*, 118–20; Cullen and Bentley, "Toxicity of Trimethylarsine."

31. Cullen and Bentley, "Toxicity of Trimethylarsine," 14.

32. Cullen, *Is Arsenic an Aphrodisiac?*, 145–61. Cullen gives a good summary of the controversy with numerous references. Examples of the substantial literature on the question of arsenic poisoning as a cause of Napoleon's death include Sten Forshufvud, *Who Killed Napoleon?* (London: Hutchinson, 1962); A. C. D. Leslie and Hamilton Smith, "Napoleon Bonaparte's Exposure to Arsenic During 1816," *Archives of Toxicology* 41 (1978): 163–67; David E. H. Jones and Kenneth W. D. Ledingham, "Arsenic in Napoleon's Wallpaper," *Nature* 299 (1982): 626–28; J. T. Hindmarsh and P. F. Corso, "The Death of Napoleon Bonaparte: A Critical Review of the Cause," *Journal of the History of Medicine and Allied Sciences* 53 (1998): 201–18.

33. Cullen, *Is Arsenic an Aphrodisiac?*, 88–89; "Clare Luce's Illness is Traced to Arsenic Dust in Rome Villa," *New York Times*, July 17, 1956.

34. Kari Konkola, "More Than a Coincidence? The Arrival of Arsenic and the Disappearance of Plague in Early Modern Europe," *Journal of the History of Medicine and Allied Sciences* 47 (1992): 186–209.

35. James Whorton, *Before* Silent Spring, 20–25. The quotation is on page 24–25.

36. Ibid., 32–33.

37. J. F. McDiarmid Clark, "Eleanor Ormerod (1828–1901) as an Economic Entomologist: 'Pioneer of Purity Even More than of Paris Green,'" *British Journal for the History of Science* 25 (1992): 431–52.

38. Ibid., 446–47. The quotation from Omerod is taken from page 447.

39. On the Manchester beer poisonings and the Royal Commission, see Whorton, *Before* Silent Spring, 82–88 and Cullen, *Is Arsenic an Aphrodisiac?*, 120–24.

40. Whorton, *Before* Silent Spring, 133–63.

41. John R. Abernathy, "Role of Arsenical Chemicals in Agriculture," in *Arsenic: Industrial, Biomedical, Environmental Perspectives*, ed. William H. Lederer and Robert J. Fensterheim (New York: Van Nostrand Reinhold, 1983), 57–60; John C. Alden, "The Continuing Need for Inorganic Arsenical Pesticides, in ibid., 63–9;

Cullen, *Is Arsenic an Aphrodisiac?*, 75–8; "Organic Arsenicals," Environmental Protection Agency, http://www.epa.gov/oppsrrd1/reregistration/organic_arsenicals_fs.html.

42. Whorton, *Arsenic Century*, 153–55; Meharg, *Venomous Earth*, 87–9. The quotation from *Puck* is on page 88.

43. Whorton, *Arsenic Century*, 160–68; Ian F. Jones, "Arsenic and the Bradford Poisonings of 1858," *Pharmaceutical Journal* 265 (2000): 938–39.

44. Whorton, *Arsenic Century*, 146–48.

45. European Food Safety Authority Panel on Contaminants in the Food Chain (CONTAM), "Scientific Opinion on Arsenic in Food," *EFSA Journal* 7 (2009): 1351; http://www.efsa.europa.eu.

46. C. E. Anderson, "Arsenicals as Feed Additives for Poultry and Swine," in *Arsenic: Perspectives*, ed. Lederer and Fensterheim, 89–97; Bette Hileman, "Arsenic in Chicken Production," *Chemical and Engineering News* 85, no. 15 (April 9, 2007); 34–35; Tom Pelton, "Lobbying by Poultry Industry in Maryland Keeps Arsenic in Chicken Feed," Bay Daily (Chesapeake Bay Foundation blog), March 23, 2011, http://cbf.typepad.com/bay_daily/2011/03/23; David Wallinga, *Playing Chicken: Avoiding Arsenic in Your Meat* (Minneapolis: Institute for Agriculture and Trade Policy, 2006).

47. Barry R. Blakely, Edward G. Clark, and Rob Fairley, "Roxarsone (3-Nitro-4-Hydroxyphenylarsonic Acid) Poisoning in Pigs," *Canadian Journal of Veterinary Medicine* 31 (1990): 385–87; Yan-xia Li and Tong-bin Chen,"Concentrations of Additive Arsenic in Beijing Pig Feeds and the Residues in Pig Manure," *Resources, Conservation and Recycling* 45 (2005): 356–67.

48. Richard Gray and Alastair Jamieson, "Arsenic and Toxic Metals found in Baby Foods," *London Telegraph*, April 9, 2011; Karin Ljung, Brita Palm, Margaretha Grandér, and Marie Vahter, "High Concentrations of Essential and Toxic Elements in Infant Formulas and Infant Foods a Matter of Concern," *Food Chemistry* 127 (2011): 943–51.

49. Whorton, *Arsenic Century*, 321–23.

50. The discussion of arsenic in drinking water is based on Meharg, *Venomous Earth*, 2–35, 158–83 (the quotation is on page 2); Cullen, *Is Arsenic an Aphrodisiac?*, 349–97.

51. The next chapter cites some of the extensive literature on arsenic eating. Here I will cite just one historical overview: Gudrun Przygoda, Jörg Feldmann, and William R. Cullen, "The Arsenic Eaters of Styria: A Different Picture of People Who Were Chronically Exposed to Arsenic," *Applied Organometallic Chemistry* 15 (2001): 457–62.

52. James F. Johnston, *The Chemistry of Common Life*, 4th ed., vol. 2 (New York: D. Appleton, 1855), 171–72.

53. Kenneth H. Winn, "Arsenic Eaters in the Nineteenth Century," *Gateway* 29 (2009): 74–83; Whorton, *Arsenic Century*, 270–76.

54. Arthur Kallet and F. J. Schlink, *100,000,000 Guinea Pigs* (New York: Grosset and Dunlap, 1933), 94, 134–35.

55. Winn, "Arsenic Eaters," 75.

56. "Fashionable Suicide," *Punch* 56 (1869): 256.

57. Winn, "Arsenic Eaters," 79–81.

58. On the poison maiden, see Richard Swiderski, *Poison Eaters: Snakes, Opium,
     Arsenic, and the Lethal Show* (Boca Raton, FL: Universal-Publishers, 2010), 23–37;
     and Norman Mosley Penzer, *Poison-damsels and Other Essays in Folklore and
     Anthropology* (New York: Arno, 1980, reprint of 1952 edition), 3–74.

59. On the history of wood preservation, see Mark Aldrich, "From Forest
     Conservation to Market Preservation: Invention and Diffusion of Wood-
     Preserving Technology, 1880–1939," *Technology and Culture* 47 (2006): 311–40;
     Michael H. Freeman, Todd F. Shupe, Richard P. Vlosky, and H. M. Barnes, "Past,
     Present, and Future of the Wood Preservation Industry," *Forest Products Journal* 53
     (2003): 8–14; Seymour S. Black, "Historical Review," in *Disinfection, Sterilization,
     and Preservation*, ed. Seymour S. Black, 5th ed. (Philadelphia: Lippincott Williams
     and Wilkins, 2001), 3–17; David Aston, "Copper/Chrome/Arsenic (CCA) Wood
     Preservatives and Their Application to Timber in the Tropics," in *Preservation of
     Timber in the Tropics*, ed. G. W. Findlay (Dordrecht: Nijhof and Junk, 1985), 141–55;
     Brian Ridout, *Timber Decay in Buildings: The Conservation Approach to Treatment*
     (London: E & FN Spon, 2000), 102; Cullen, *Is Arsenic an Aphrodisiac?*, 67–72.

60. Cullen, *Is Arsenic an Aphrodisiac?*, 66–72 (the quotation is on page 69); Greg Kidd,
     "CCA-Treated Lumber Poses Danger from Arsenic and Chromium," *Pesticides and
     You* 21, no. 3 (2001): 13–15.

61. Cullen, *Is Arsenic an Aphrodisiac?*, 67–74; Kidd, "CCA-Treated Lumber;" Mojgan
     Nejad and Paul Cooper, "Coatings to Reduce Wood Preservative Leaching,"
     Environmental Science and Technology 44 (2010): 6162–66; J. R., "Skin Proves Poor
     Portal for Arsenic in Treated Wood," *Science News* 166, no. 4 (July 24, 2004): 62.

62. Cullen, *Is Arsenic an Aphrodisiac?*, 324–25; Badal Kumar Mandal and Kazuo T.
     Suzuki, "Arsenic Round the World: A Review," *Talanta* 58 (2002); 201–35; K. W.
     Nelson, "Industrial Contributions of Arsenic in the Environment," *Environmental
     Health Perspectives* 19 (1977): 31–34; and C. S. Weiss, E. J. Parks, and F. E.
     Brinkman, "Speciation of Arsenic in Fossil Fuels and Their Conversion Process
     Fluids," in Lederer and Fensterheim, eds., *Arsenic: Perspectives*, 309–26.

63. Timothy LeCain, "The Limits of 'Eco-Efficiency:' Arsenic Pollution and the
     Cottrell Electrical Precipitator in the U. S. Copper Smelting Industry,"
     Environmental History 5 (2000): 336–51. The quotation is on page 340.

64. Ibid., 340.

65. Frederic L. Quivik, "The Tragic Montana Career of Dr. D. E. Salmon," *Montana:
     The Magazine of Western History* 57, no. 1 (Spring 2007): 32–47. The quotation is on
     page 43.

66. The discussion of the Anaconda incident is based on LeCain, "Limits;" Quivik,
     "Tragic Montana Career;" and Gordon Morris Bakken, "Was There Arsenic in
     the Air? Anaconda versus the Farmers of Deer Lodge Valley," *Montana: The
     Magazine of Western History* 41, no. 3 (Summer 1991): 30–41.

67. Cullen, *Is Arsenic an Aphrodisiac?*, 319–22. The quotation is on page 319.

68. For examples of scientists challenging what they believe to be unreasonable fears
     about the dangers of arsenic, including challenging its carcinogenicity, see
     Douglas V. Frost, "The Arsenic Problems," *Advances in Experimental Medicine and*

Biology 91 (1977): 259–79; Ralph A. Zingaro, "Arsenic—A Classic Example of Chemophobia," *Environment International* 19 (1993): 167–78.

5. What Kills Can Cure: Arsenic in Medicine

1. Henry E. Sigerist, ed., *Four Treatises of Theophrastus von Hohenheim, called Paracelsus, Translated from the original German* (Baltimore: Johns Hopkins University Press, 1941), 21. For a treatise on Paracelsus's life and work, see Walter Pagel, *Paracelsus: An Introduction to Philosophical Medicine in the Era of the Renaissance*, 2nd ed. (Basel: Karger, 1982).

2. Meharg, *Venomous Earth*, 40–41; Cullen, *Is Arsenic an Aphrodisiac?*, 2–5; John Emsley, *The Elements of Murder: A History of Poison* (Oxford, England: Oxford University Press, 2005), 94, 104.

3. R. P. Multhauf, *The Origins of Chemistry* (London: Oldbourne, 1966), 229; Walter Sneader, *Drug Discovery: A History* (Chichester: John Wiley and Sons, 2005), 48; Erwin H. Ackerknecht, *Therapeutics from the Primitives to the 20th Century* (New York: Hafner Press, 1973), 48; Martin Levey, *The Medical Formulary or Aqrābādhīn of al-Kindī* (Madison: University of Wisconsin Press, 1966).

4. Multhauf, *Origins of Chemistry*, 201–36; Sneader, *Drug Discovery*, 48–49; John S. Haller Jr., "Therapeutic Mule: The Use of Arsenic in the Nineteenth Century Materia Medica," *Pharmacy in History* 17 (1975): 87–100.

5. Haller, "Therapeutic Mule," 88.

6. On the history of Fowler's Solution, see Haller, "Therapeutic Mule"; Whorton, *Arsenic Century*, 229–41; Cullen, *Is Arsenic an Aphrodisiac?*, 13–19; "Dr. Thomas Fowler''s Solution," *British Medical Journal* (1922): 115–16; H. A. Langenhan, *Liquor Potassii Arsenitis* (Madison: University of Wisconsin, 1918).

7. Thomas Fowler, *Medical Reports on the Effects of Arsenic in the Cure of Agues, Remitting Fevers, and Periodic Headachs* (London: J. Johnson, 1786), 108–9.

8. Fowler, *Medical Reports*, 105–9 (quotation on page 106); Whorton, *Arsenic Century*, 234–35.

9. Cullen, *Is Arsenic an Aphrodisiac?*, 16–17; Whorton, *Arsenic Century*, 235–36; Langerhan, *Liquor*, 7–8.

10. Haller, "Therapeutic Mule," 89–92.

11. Whorton, *Arsenic Century*, 236–39; Haller, "Therapeutic Mule," 98.

12. Committee on Medical and Biologic Effects of Environmental Pollutants, National Research Council, *Arsenic: Medical and Biologic Effects of Environmental Pollutants* (Washington, DC: National Academy of Sciences, 1977), 174; Stanley Scheindlin, "The Duplicitous Nature of Inorganic Arsenic," *Molecular Interventions* 5 (2005): 60–64; H. Falk, G. G. Caldwell, K. G. Ishak, L. B. Thomas, and H. Popper, "Arsenic-Related Hepatic Angiosarcoma," *American Journal of Industrial Medicine* 2 (1981); 43–50; Michael L. Kasper, Lynn Schoenfield, Robert L. Strom, and Athanasios Theologides, "Hepatic Angiosarcoma and Bronchioloalveolar Carcinoma Induced by Fowler's Solution," *Journal of the American Medical Association* 252 (1984): 3407–8.

13. Whorton, *Arsenic Century*, 240.

14. For biographical information on Tschudi, see Paul-Emile Schazmann, *Johann Jakob von Tschudi: Forscher, Arzt, Diplomat* (Glarus: Baeschlin, 1956); Friedrich Ratzel, "Tschudi, Johann Jakob von," in *Allgemeine Deutsche Biographie*, vol. 38 (Leipzig: Duncker and Humblot, 1894), 749–52.

15. J. J. von Tschudi, "Über die Giftesser," *Wiener Medizinische Wochenschrift* 1 (1851): 454–55. An English translation of a French version of this paper and a follow-up paper by Tschudi from 1853 were published under the title of "Arsenic Eaters" in the *Boston Medical and Surgical Journal* 51 (1854): 189–95. The quotation is taken from page 190. Another English translation of most of Tschudi's 1851 paper appeared in the article by W. B. Kesteven, "On Arsenic Eating," *Association Medical Journal*, 3–4 (1856): 721–22.

16. "Arsenic Eaters," *Boston Medical and Surgical Journal*, 1854; Charles Boner, "Poison-Eaters," *Chamber's Journal of Popular Literature, Science and Arts* 5 (1856): 90; James F. Johnston, *The Chemistry of Common Life*, 4th ed., vol. 2 (New York: D. Appleton, 1855), 166–72.

17. W. B. Kesteven, "On Arsenic Eating," *Association Medical Journal* 3–4 (1856): 721–22, 757–59, 808–12.

18. Charles Heisch, "On the Arsenic-Eaters of Styria," *Pharmaceutical Journal*, second series, 1 (1860): 556–60; Henry Enfield Roscoe, "On the Alleged Practice of Arsenic-Eating in Styria," *Memoirs of the Literary and Philosophical Society of Manchester*, third series, 1 (1862): 208–21 (quotation on page 221).

19. Roscoe, "Arsenic-Eating," 214–15.

20. Craig Maclagan, "On the Arsenic-Eaters of Styria," *Edinburgh Medical Journal* 10 (1864): 200–207.

21. Craig Maclagan, "Arsenic-Eaters of Styria," *Edinburgh Medical Journal* 21 (1875): 526–28; "The Arsenic Eaters of Styria," *British Medical Journal* 2 (1875): 437.

22. H. E. Roscoe, *A Treatise on Chemistry*, 3rd ed., vol. 1 (London: Macmillan, 1905), 684–85; Robert W. MacKenna, "The Toleration of Arsenic," *British Medical Journal* 1 (1901): 85.

23. M. Cloetta, "Ueber die Ursache der Angewöhnung an Arsenik," *Archiv für experimentelle Pathologie und Pharmakologie* 54 (1906): 196-205; Thomas W. Clarkson, "Inorganic and Organometal Pesticides," in *Handbook of Pesticide Toxicology: Principles*, ed. Robert Irving Krieger, 2nd ed., vol. 1 (San Diego: Academic Press, 2001), 1357–1428; Erich W. Schwartze, "The So-Called Habituation to 'Arsenic': Variation in the Toxicity of Arsenious Oxide," *Journal of Pharmacology and Experimental Therapeutics* 20 (1922): 181–203; Erich W. Schwartze and James C. Munch, "So-Called Habituation to 'Arsenic,'": 351–60 (quotation is on page 360); F. L. Campbell, "On the Possibility of Development of Tolerance to Arsenic by Individual Insects," *Journal of Economic Entomology* 19 (1926): 516–22. The quotation is on page 521.

24. See, for example, J. R. Shaw, B. Jackson, S. Stanton, J. W. Hamilton, and B. A. Stanton, ""The Influence of Exposure History on Arsenic Accumulation in the Killfish, *Fundulus Heteroclitus*," *Environmental Toxicology and Chemistry* 26 (2007): 2407–9; Elizabeth H. Romach et al., "Studies on the Mechanism of Arsenic-Induced Self Tolerance Developed in Liver Epithelial Cells through Continuous Low-Level Arsenite Exposure," *Toxicological Sciences* 54 (2000): 500–8; Eduardo M. Brambila, William E. Achanzar, Wei Qu, Mukta M. Webber, and Michael P.

Waalkes, "Chronic Arsenic-Exposed Human Prostrate Epithelial Cells Exhibit Stable Arsenic Tolerance: Mechanistic Implications of Altered Cellular Glutathione and Glutathione S-Transferase," *Toxicology and Applied Pharmacology* 183 (2002): 99–107; Bhaskar Rao Bondada and Lena Qiying Ma, "Tolerance of Heavy Metals in Vascular Plants: Arsenic Hyperaccumulation by Chinese Brake Fern (*Pterzs Vzttatal*)," in *Pteridology in the New Millennium*, ed. S. Chandra and M. Srivastava (Dordrecht: Kluwer, 2003), 397–420.

25. Cullen, *Is Arsenic an Aphrodisiac?*, 12.

26. Ibid., 9–10. The quotation is on page 10.

27. Ibid., 10–11.

28. Dietmar Steverding, "The History of African Trypanosomiasis," *Parasites and Vectors* 1 (2008): 3 (available only online at http://www.ncbi.nlm.nih.gov/pmc /articles/PMC2270819/).

29. Dietmar Steverding, "The Development of Drugs for Treatment of Sleeping Sickness: A Historical Review," *Parasites and Vectors* 3 (2010): 15 (available only online at http://www.ncbi.nlm.nih.gov/pmc/articles/PMC2848007/); James Braid, "The Bite of the Tsetse Fly: Arsenic Suggested as a Remedy," *British Medical Journal* 1 (1858): 135; and David Livingstone, "Arsenic as a Remedy for the Tsetse Bite," *British Medical Journal* 1 (1868): 360–61.

30. Steverding, "Development of Drugs"; H. Wolferstan Thomas, "Some Experiments in the Treatment of Trypanosomiasis," *British Medical Journal* 1 (1905): 1140–43. The quotation is on page 1140.

31. Steverding, "Development of Drugs;" Wolfgang U. Eckart, "The Colony as Laboratory: German Sleeping Sickness Campaigns in German East Africa and in Togo, 1900–1914," *History and Philosophy of the Life Sciences* 24 (2002): 69–89.

32. For biographical information on Ehrlich, see Martha Marquardt, *Paul Ehrlich* (New York: Henry Schuman, 1953), 59–60; Ernst Bäunler, *Paul Ehrlich: Scientist for Life*, translated by Grant Edwards (New York: Holmes and Meier, 1984).

33. On Ehrlich's chemotherapy and the development of Salvarsan, see John Parascandola, "The Theoretical Basis of Paul Ehrlich's Chemotherapy," *Journal of the History of Medicine and Allied Sciences* 36 (1981): 19–43.

34. On this incident, see Baümler, *Paul Ehrlich*, 202–10 (quotation on page 202–3); Marquardt, *Paul Ehrlich*, 235–38.

35. John Patrick Swann, "Arthur Tatum, Parke-Davis, and the Discovery of Mapharsen as an Antisyphilitic Agent," *Journal of the History of Medicine and Allied Sciences* 40 (1985): 167–87.

36. John Parascandola, *Sex, Sin, and Science: A History of Syphilis in America* (Westport, CT: Praeger, 2008), 79–80.

37. Parascandola, *Sex, Sin, and Science*, 119–128; John Parascandola, "Quarantining Women: Venereal Disease Rapid Treatment Centers in World War II America," *Bulletin of the History of Medicine* 83 (2009): 431–59.

38. John Parascandola, "John Mahoney and the Introduction of Penicillin to Treat Syphilis," *Pharmacy in History* 43 (2001): 3–13.

39. Shearjashub Spooner, *Guide to Sound Teeth, or a Popular Treatise on the Teeth*, 2nd ed. (New York: Collins, Keese and Company, 1838), 116.

40. Whorton, *Arsenic Century*, 259.

41. On the history of arsenic in dentistry, see John M. Hyson Jr., "A History of Arsenic in Dentistry," *Journal of the California Dental Association* 35 (2007): 135–39; Whorton, *Arsenic Century*, 258–60; Cullen, *Is Arsenic an Aphrodisiac?*, 19. For a recent example of problems caused by arsenic use in dentistry, see M. S. Yavuz, G. Sims, E. K. Kaya, and M. H. Aras, "Mandibular Bone Necrosis Caused by Use of Arsenic Paste During Endodontic Treatment: Two Case Reports," *International Endodontic Journal* 41 (2008): 633–37.

42. Gordon Piller, "Leukemia—A Brief Historical Review from Ancient Times to 1950," *British Journal of Haematology* 112 (2001): 282–92; Samuel Waksman and Kenneth C. Anderson, "History of the Development of Arsenic Derivatives in Cancer Therapy," *The Oncologist* 6 (2001): supplement 3–10.

43. Waksman and Anderson, "Arsenic Derivatives," 4.

44. Elisabeth Rosenthal, "Chairman Mao's Cure for Cancer," *New York Times Magazine*, May 6, 2001, 70–73. The quotation is on page 70.

45. Ibid., 73.

46. Waxman and Anderson, "Arsenic Derivatives;" Jun Zhu, Zhu Chen, Valérie Lallemand-Breitenbach, and Hugues de Thé, "How Acute Promyelocytic Leukaemia Revived Arsenic," *Nature Reviews Cancer* 2 (2002): 705–14; and Cullen, *Is Arsenic an Aphrodisiac?*, 20–22.

47. Andrew Wilson and H. O. Schild, eds., *Clark's Applied Pharmacology*, 8th ed. (Philadelphia: Blakiston, 1952), 3.

48. On the history of homeopathy, see John S. Haller Jr., *The History of American Homeopathy: From Rational Medicine to Holistic Health Care* (New Brunswick, NJ: Rutgers University Press, 2009); Harris Coulter, *Divided Legacy: A History of the Schism in Medical Thought*, four volumes (Berkeley, CA: North Atlantic Books, 1982–96).

49. Constantine Hering, *The Guiding Symptoms of Our Materia Medica*, vol. 2 (Philadelphia: American Homeopathic Publishing Society, 1880), 31–97.

50. Stephen B. Kayne, *Homeopathic Pharmacy: Theory and Practice*, 2nd ed. (Edinburgh: Elsevier Churchill Livingstone, 2006), 340.

51. For example, see D. Chakraborti et al., "Arsenic Toxicity from Homeopathic Treatment," *Journal of Toxicology and Clinical Toxicology* 41 (2003): 963–67.

52. P. Mallick, J. Chakrabarti Mallick, B. Guha, and A. R. Khuda-Bukhsh, "Ameliorating Effect of Microdoses of a Potentized Homeopathic Drug, Arsenicum Album, on Arsenic-Induced Toxicity in Mice," *BMC Complementary and Alternative Medicine*, 2003, http://www.biomedcentral.com/1472-6882/3/7; Anisur Rahman et al., "Can Homeopathic Arsenic Remedy Combat Arsenic Poisoning in Humans Exposed to Groundwater Arsenic Contamination?: A Preliminary Report on First Human Trial," *Evidence-Based Complementary and Alternative Medicine* 2 (2005): 537–48; Cullen, *Is Arsenic an Aphrodisiac?*, 14.

53. Richard J. Ko, "Adulterants in Asian Patent Medicines," *New England Journal of Medicine* 339 (1998): 847; Robert B. Saper et al., "Lead, Mercury, and Arsenic in US- and Indian-Manufactured Ayurvedic Medicines Sold via the Internet," *Journal of the American Medical Association* 300 (2008): 915–23; E. Ernst, "Heavy Metals in Traditional Indian Remedies," *European Journal of Clinical Pharmacology*

57 (2002): 891–96; Kelli Cooper et al., "Public Health Risks from Heavy Metals and Metalloids Present in Traditional Chinese Medicines," *Journal of Toxicology and Environmental Health, Part A* 70 (2007): 1694–99; M. J. Martena et al., "Monitoring of Mercury, Arsenic, and Lead in Traditional Asian Herbal Preparations on the Dutch Market and Estimation of Associated Risks," *Food Additives and Contaminants, Part A* 27 (2010): 190–205.

54. C. H. Tay and C. S. Seah, "Arsenic-Poisoning from Anti-Asthmatic Herbal Preparations," *Medical Journal of Australia* 2 (1975): 424–28.

55. S. S. Wong , K. C. Tan, and C. L. Koh, "Cutaneous Manifestations of Chronic Arsenicism: Review of Seventeen Cases," *Journal of the American Academy of Dermatology* 38 (1998): 179–85; John Kew et al., "Arsenic and Mercury Intoxication Due to Indian Ethnic Remedies," *British Medical Journal* 306 (1993): 506–7.

Index

Accum, Frederick, 69
Addington, Anthony, 9–10
Agricola, Georgius (Georg Bauer), 84
Alchemist, The (Johnson) 73
Anaconda Copper Mining Company, 141–43
Animal feed, arsenic in, 130–31
Archer-Gilligan, Amy, 48
Armstrong murder case, 30–33: Armstrong, Herbert Rowse, 30–33; Armstrong, Katherine Mary Friend, 30–31, 32, 33; Martin, Oswald, 31–32, 33
arsenic: in atmosphere, 110, 140–43; building immunity to, 60, 61, 70–71 (*see also* arsenic eaters of Styria); concentration in earth's crust, 2; contamination of drinking water in Bangladesh and West Bengal, 2, 132–34, 169–70; commercial use becomes widespread, 109–10; detection of, 9–12 (*see also* Marsh test, Reinsch test); in earth's crust, 2, 110; ease of obtaining, 8; as element, 2; famous murder cases, 16–46 (*see also under names of individual cases*); gastrointestinal effects of, 1, 61; most common poison in England, 7–8; as murder weapon in antiquity, 5–6; as murder weapon in 15th-18th centuries, 6–7; as murder weapon in 19th century, 7–8 (*see also under names of individual cases*); origin of word, 1; physical properties, 1, 5; preservation of human bodies by, 62 (*see also* embalming: arsenic in); reasons for popularity as poison, 1, 5; restrictions on sale, 12–15; use to promote general health, 22, 26 (*see also* arsenic eaters of Styria; Styrian defense)
Arsenic and Gold (Atkey), 63
Arsenic and Old Lace (Kesserling), 78
Arsenic and Old Paint (Lind), 63
arsenic-based bacteria, 3
arsenic eaters of Styria, 26, 56, 60, 63, 70–71, 134, 151–56 (*see also* Styrian defense)
arsenic flypaper, 25–26, 28–30, 38, 61, 109
arsenic (arsenious) oxide. See arsenic trioxide

arsenic sulfides. *See* orpiment; realgar
arsenic trioxide (arsenic oxide), 1, 3, 5, 8, 63, 86, 87, 106, 121, 124, 129, 130, 134, 137, 143, 146, 149, 154, 164, 166, 167
Arsenicum album, 169, 170
arsenophobia, 123, 144
arsine, 10, 60, 103, 107, 121
artificial flowers, arsenic in, 88–89, 109, 111, 114, 117
Asarco, 143
As a Thief in the Night (Freeman), 58–59
Atkey, Bertram, *Arsenic and Gold*, 63

Bartrip, Peter, 14, 89, 90–91, 109, 112, 119
Bécouer, Jean-Baptiste, 93
Blackstock, Terri, *Shadow of Doubt*, 62
Blandy murder case, 9–10; Blandy, Mary, 9–10; Cranstoun, William, 9–10
Borgia family, 6
Bureau of Chemistry, United States Department of Agriculture, 127–28, 155
Busch, Charles, *Die, Mommy, Die!*, 79

candles, arsenic-containing: as murder weapon in fiction, 59, 60–61; manufacture of, 59
Canterbury Tales, The (Chaucer), 73
Case of the Drowsy Mosquito, The (Gardner), 61-62
Challenger, Frederick, 122
Chaucer, Geoffrey, *The Canterbury Tales*, 73
chemical warfare: American University Experiment Station, 48; arsenic used in, 47–49; British anti-Lewisite, 49; Catholic University of America, 47; Chemical Warfare Service, 47; contamination of sites by chemical agents, 50–51; Griffin, John, 47; human experimentation with chemical agents, 50; Lewsite, 48–49; Lewis, Winifred, Lee, 47–49; Nieuwland, Julius Aloyius, 47–48; prohibitions on use of, 47, 49, 50; in World War I, 47–49

Children's Employment Commission, 89, 90, 91

Christie, Agatha, 64–68; *Easy to Kill*, 66; *Funerals are Fatal*, 68; *The Mirror Crack'd*, 68; *The Mysterious Affair at Styles*, 64; *They Came to Baghdad*, 66; *Third Girl*, 68; *The Tuesday Club Murders*, 65–66; *What Mrs. McGillicuddy Saw*, 66

Christison, Robert, 21, 153

chromated copper arsenate (CCA), 107, 137–40; in playground equipment, 139 (*see also* wood preservative: use of arsenic as)

cinchona bark, 148, 149

Cloetta, Max, 155

Clothing, use of arsenic in, 109, 110, 111, 117, 119

Collins, Wilkie, 54–57; *The Law and the Lady*, 54–57, 55; *The Moonstone*, 54

Copper arsenate, 130, 147

cosmetic, use of arsenic as, 21, 26, 109, 134–37, 152, 153; defense in murder trial, 21, 22, 26, 56 (*see also* arsenic eaters of Styria; Styrian defense)

Croydon murders, 33–37; Duff, Grace Sidney, 34, 35, 36–37; Duff, Edmund, 34, 36; Elwell, Robert, 34, 35, 36; Sidney, Tom, 34, 36–37; Sidney, Vera, 34, 35, 36; Sidney, Violet, 35–36

Cullen, William, 2, 94, 121, 122–23, 138, 143, 156

d'Aubray, Madeleine-Marguérite, 7

DDT (dichlorodiphenyltrichloroethane), 106, 124, 128

Death Lights a Candle (Taylor), 60–61

dentistry, arsenic in, 164–65

detective fiction: arsenic in, 53–73; origins of, 53–54; use of actual features of arsenic poisoning in, 56, 57

Devons Great Consols mine, 87, 114

Dickens, Charles, 54

Doherty, Paul, *The Queen of the Night*, 62

Doyle, Arthur Conan, 54

Draper, Frank, 117–18

Dr. Campbell's Safe Arsenic Complexion Wafers, 135, 136

drinking water, arsenic in, 2, 132–34, 169–70

Dupin, C. Auguste, 53–54

Easy to Kill (Christie), 66

Ehrlich, Paul, 158–163

embalming, 98–105; American Civil War, 100–104; arsenic used in, 62, 63, 99–105; chemical preservatives first used in, 99; hazards of arsenic use to embalmers and others who handled human remains, 102–5; interference of arsenic use in criminal investigations, 100, 102–3, 103–4

emerald green. See Paris green

Emsley, John, 1, 27

Environment, arsenic in, 109–144. *See also under* specific headings, such as *drinking water: arsenic in*

Faulkner, William, 80–81

Fiction, arsenic in, 53–82. *See also* individual authors and titles

Flaubert, Gustave (*Madame Bovary*), 75–77, 79

food, arsenic in, 109, 111, 117, 119, 128–29, 130–31; baby food, 131; beer (*see* Manchester beer poisonings); candy, 109, 117, 128–29; chicken, 130–31; pesticide residues (*see* pesticides, arsenic); wine, 129

Fowler's solution, 135, 147–51, 165, 166

Fowler, Thomas, 147–49

free enterprise and regulation of arsenic, 111, 118

Freeman, R. Austin (*As a Thief in the Night*), 57–59

Funerals are Fatal (Christie), 68

Gannal, J. N., 95, 99, 103

Gardner, Erle Stanley (*The Case of the Drowsy Mosquito*), 61

Gilman, Charlotte Perkins, 74

Goolrick, Robert (*A Reliable Wife*), 81

Gosio, Bartolomeo, 121–22; Gosio gas (trimethylarsine), 122, 123; Gosio's disease, 122

The Green of the Period (anonymous), 74, 75, 115

Gustav Adolf Lutheran Church, arsenic poisonings at, 45–46; Bondeson, Daniel, 45–46; Bondeson, Norma, 45–46; Kelley, Peter, 46

Guy, William, 89

Hammett, Dashiel, 61

Hahnemann, Samuel, 168-69

Hassall, Arthur Hill, 88, 114, 115, 128

Hill, G. N., 149, 150

Hinds, William, 113

Hippocrates, 145, 146

Holmes, Sherlock, 53–54

Holmes, Thomas, 100

homeopathy, arsenic in, 82, 168–170

Hough, Walter, 94, 95

Housman, A. E., 71

Hungary, arsenic poisonings in. *See* Tiszakürt, arsenic poisonings in village of

If I'd Killed Him When I Met Him (McCrumb), 63

Jackson, Shirley (*We Have Always Lived in the Castle*), 80–81

Johnson, Ben (*The Alchemist*), 73

Johnston, James F., 134–35, 152–53

Kamesan, Sonti, 137–38

Kedzie, Robert, 118–19, 120; *Shadows from the Walls of Death*, 118–19

Kesserling, Joseph (*Arsenic and Old Lace*), 78

Kesteven, W. B., 153

Knappe (Austrian physician). *See* arsenic eaters of Styria

Lafarge, Marie, murder trial, 11–12
Laveran, Charles, 157–58
Law and The Lady, The (Collins), 54–57; Brinton, Valeria, 54–56; Macallan, Sara, 54–57, Macallan, Eustace, 54–56
lead arsenate, 106, 123, 124, 127, 128
leukemia, use of arsenic in treatment of. *See* medicine, arsenic as: in cancer treatment
Lewisite. *See under* chemical warfare
Lewis, Winifred Lee, 47–49
Lind, Hailey (*Arsenic and Old Paint*), 63
Livingstone, David, 157
Lloyd, Phoebe, 97–98
London purple (monocalcium arsenite), 106, 124
Lord, Henry, 90–91
Luce, Clare Boothe, 123–24
Lyons, Mary E. (*The Poison Place*), 82

Maclagan, Craig, 154–55
Madame Bovary (Flaubert), 75–78, 77; Bovary, Charles, 76, 78; Bovary, Emma, 75–78
Manchester beer poisonings, 126–27
Marsh, James, 10
Marsh test for arsenic, 10–12, 11, 57, 58, 72, 121
Mason, Perry, 62
Maybrick murder case, 23–27; Chandler, Caroline Holbrook, 23–24; Maybrick, Florence, 23–27; Maybrick, James, 24–26
Marple, Jane, 65–66, 68
McCrumb, Sharyn (*If I'd Killed Him When I Met Him*), 63
McCurdy, Elmer, 102
de Medici, Catherine, 6
medicine, arsenic in, 3, 145–71; in antiquity, 145–46; in cancer treatment, 3, 146, 165–68; in dentistry, 164–65; in dermatology, 150; in folk remedies and patent medicines, 170–71; in homeopathy, 82, 168–70; in malaria treatment, 148, 149, 156; in medieval Islam, 146; popularity in 18th and 19th centuries, 147, 150–51; as tonic, 150; in traditional Chinese medicine, 170–71; in treatment of syphilis, 161–64; in treatment of trypanosomiasis, 158–60. *See also* arsenic eaters of Styria
Meharg, Andrew, 86, 114, 133–34
Miller murder case, 43–45; Miller, Ann, 43–45; Miller, Eric, 43–44; Morgan, Chris, 43–44
Miller, Lillian, 97–98
mining and smelting, arsenic in, 83–88, 132, 140–43; in antiquity, 83–84; contamination of drinking water, 132; Devons Great Consols mine, 87; hazards to workers, 84, 86–88; in Middle Ages and Renaissance, 84; Paracelsus on, 84; Ramazzini on, 86; as source of air pollution, 140–43; Thackrah on, 86.
Mineral green. *See* Scheele's green
Minsterborough (Sandwith), 74

The Mirror Crack'd (Christie), 68
Mithridates, 71
Monvoisin, Catherine Deshayes, 7
Morris, Pat, 96
Morris, William, 87, 114–15
murder, use of arsenic for. *See the following subheadings under* arsenic: famous murder cases; as murder weapon in antiquity; as murder weapon in 15th–18th centuries; as murder weapon in 19th century
Mysterious Affair at Styles, The (Christie), 64

Napoleon, arsenic as possible cause of death, 123
Nrigau, Jerome, 83

Omerod, Eleanor, 126
Orfila, Matthieu, 12, 13
orpiment, 3, 73, 92, 145, 146, 154, 155

paint, arsenic in. *See* pigment, use of arsenic as
Paracelsus, 84, 145, 146–47
Paris green (copper acetoarsenite), 59, 60, 88, 90, 92, 106, 110, 118, 124, 125, 126
Peale, Charles Wilson, 82, 97
Peale, Raphaelle, 82, 97–98
pesticides, arsenic, 106, 124–28, 143; risks to farm workers, 106, 124; hazards to consumers of residues on produce, 125, 127–28; as weed killer, 33, 57, 128
Phar Lap, possible arsenic poisoning of, 156
Philadelphia poison ring, 40–43; Alfonsi, Ferdinand, 40–41; Alfonsi, Stella, 40–41; Arena, Anna, 40–41; Arena, Joseph, 40–41; Bolber, Morris, 40–43; Myer, George, 41–42; Petrillo, Herman, 40–43; Petrillo, Paul, 40–43
pigment, use of arsenic as, 2, 89–92, 109, 110, 111, 112, 113–21, 123–24, 128–29, 143; hazards to artists and painters, 91–92; hazards to factory workers, 90–91. *See also* London purple; Paris green; Scheele's green; wallpaper, arsenic in
Poe, Edgar Allen, 53–54
Poirot, Hercule, 65, 66–67
poison maiden, legend of, 136–37; "Rappaccini's Daughter" (Nathaniel Hawthorne), 137
poison, as woman's weapon, 8, 39, 68
Poison Place, The (Lyons), 82
poison widows. *See* Philadelphia poison ring
preservation of corpses by arsenic, 62, 99. *See also* embalming

Queen of the Night, The (Doherty), 62

Ramazzini, Bernadino, 84–86, 91–92
rapid treatment methods for syphilis, 163–64
rat poison, arsenic as, 8, 17, 21, 57, 61, 76, 80, 124, 132, 147; possible factor in disappearance of plague from Europe, 124, 147

realgar, 3, 73, 92, 145, 146
Reinsch, Hugo, 12
Reinsch test for arsenic, 12, 59
Rice, William, 113
Reliable Wife, A (Goolrick), 81
Roscoe, Henry Enfield, 153–54, 155
roxarsone (3-nitro-4-hydroxyphenylarsonic acid), 130–31
Russell, Niamh, 82

Saha, K. C., 133
Salvarsan (606), 161–63
Sandwith, Humphrey (*Minsterborough*), 74
Sayers, Dorothy, 27, 68–73; *Strong Poison*, 27, 68–71
Scheele's green (copper arsenite), 59, 66, 88, 89, 92, 110, 111, 113, 121
Schwartze, Erich, 155
Schwendeman, Bruce, 96–97
Seddon murder case, 27–30; Barrow, Eliza, 27–30; Seddon, Frederick, 27–30, 29; Seddon, Maggie, 28–29; Seddon, Margaret, 27–28, 30
Shadow of Doubt (Blackstock), 62–63
Shadows from the Walls of Death (Kedzie), 118–19
sheep dressing (dipping), hazards of arsenic use to workers, 105
Smith murder case, 18–23; L'Angelier, Pierre Emile, 18–23; Minnoch, William, 19–20; Smith, Madeleine, 18–23
Spara, Hieronyma, 6
Styrian defense, 26, 56. *See also* arsenic eaters of Styria
Sweeney murder case, 16–18; Broadnax, Lydia, 16–17; Brown, Michael, 16–17; Sweeney, George Wythe, 16–18; Wythe, George, 16–18

taxidermy, arsenic in, 82, 92–98; for preserving museum specimens, 94–95; hazards to taxidermists and museum workers and visitors, 94–98. *See also* Peale, Raphaelle
Taylor, Alfred Swaine, 14, 111, 113, 115, 153
Taylor, Phoebe Atwood (*Death Lights a Candle*), 60
Thackrah, Charles Turner, 86, 92
They Came to Baghdad (Christie), 66
Third Girl (Christie), 68
Thomas, H. Wolferstan, 158
Thorndyke, John Evelyn, 57–59

Tiszakürt, arsenic poisonings in village of, 37–39; Fazekas, Zsuzsanna, 37, 38–39. *See also* poison, as woman's weapon
Toffana, Giulia, 6
tolerance to arsenic. *See* arsenic eaters of Stryria
toys, use of arsenic in, 109, 110, 111, 117
Tranchina, G., 99, 102
Trestrail III, John Harris, 53
Tschudi, Johann Jakob von, 151–52, 153

Vane, Harriet, 69–71

wallpaper, arsenic in, 60, 63, 89–90, 109, 111, 112–23; mechanism of poisoning by, 112–13, 114, 115, 121–23; possible cause of death of Napoleon, 123; decline in popularity, 119–21
Wassmann, Karl, 162–63
Watson, Katherine, 7–8
We Have Always Lived in the Castle (Jackson), 80–81
What Mrs. McGillicuddy Saw (Christie), 66
Whimsey, Lord Peter, 69–71
Whorton, James, 59, 73, 104, 105, 109, 110, 115, 124, 129, 132, 149, 165
Wilbert, Martin, 15
white arsenic. *See* arsenic trioxide
Wolfe-Simon, Felisa, 3
Wood, Edward S., 119
wood preservative use of arsenic as, 106–7, 137–40, 143; risks to workers and consumers, 106–7; in playground equipment, 139. *See also* chromated copper arsenate (CCA)
workplace, arsenic in, 83–107; in artificial flower trade, 88-89; in embalming, 98–105; in mining and smelting, 83–88; in miscellaneous occupations, 105–7; in paint and wallpaper manufacture and use, 89–92; in taxidermy, 92–98
women and poison. *See* poison, as woman's weapon

yellow arsenic. *See* orpiment
"Yellow Wallpaper, The" (Gilman), 74

Zhang Tingdong, 167

About the Author

John Parascandola received his PhD in the history of science from the University of Wisconsin–Madison. In a career spanning more than forty years, he has served on the faculty of the University of Wisconsin–Madison, as chief of the History of Medicine Division of the National Library of Medicine, and as Public Health Service historian. Dr. Parascandola is the author of *The Development of American Pharmacology: John J. Abel and the Shaping of a Discipline* (1992) and *Sex, Sin and Science: A History of Syphilis in America* (2008). He is currently on the adjunct faculty of the Department of History at the University of Maryland-College Park.